S

D1601419

Death by HMO

The Jennifer Gigliello Story

by
Dorothy Rose Cancilla
as told to Richard N. Côté

Dedicated Press
Pacifica, California

S

Copyright © 1999 by Dorothy Rose Cancilla

ISBN 0-9671922-0-X

Library of Congress Catalog Card Number: 98-41967

Dedicated Press
Pacifica, California

Cover Design by Julia Gaskill
Typesetting by Barbara Kruger

All names of doctors, nurses, hospitals and attorneys have been changed. The only exceptions:

1) Kaiser Hospital, which lost the wrongful death suit filed by Jennifer Gigliello's husband and son, has been retained, and

2) Attorney, Gary Moss, from the law firm of Moss & Hought, San Francisco, who successfully pressed the case against Kaiser for the family.

In 1986, Paul Gigliello and his son, Paul Gigliello, Jr., filed a suit against Kaiser for the wrongful death of their wife and mother. On February 10, 1995, an arbitration panel awarded the plaintiffs $175,000. The maximum amount allowable under California law would have been $250,000. Kaiser did not appeal the award.

Dedication

In loving memory of my daughter, Jennifer, and my husband, Lou, whom I love and miss very much, and who together showed an enormous amount of courage and strength. Your beautiful, gentle spirits and example of love will forever live in our hearts.

And to all victims and their families who are suffering from medical neglect. Let us pray for the humility to accept that we need help and firmness of purpose to take action to get it. Let us ask for the aid of our Higher Power in striving for a better way so that we may acquire dignity and respect for all those in need. Our common welfare should come first; personal progress for the greatest number depends on unity. Let us always be ready to carry the message to others. The need is all around us if we keep ourselves alert enough to recognize it. In helping others, we also help ourselves. Sharing experiences widens one's horizons and opens new and better ways of dealing with life's problems.

There is no need to solve them alone.

In Appreciation

My heartfelt thanks go to many fine people.

First and foremost to my children Rosemarie, Vince and Cathy. Rosemarie, your unconditional love and dedication to your sister Jennifer during those critical moments has been an inspiration to us all. Vince, you stood by me at a very difficult time in my life; I could not ask for a more loving and caring son. Cathy, your determination to see that Jennifer's story is told and your continuing hard work has been admirable. Bob and Lester, my two sons-in-law, your patience and understanding through the last few years has been overwhelming. To my loving dear children, thank you. I could have never done it without you.

To my dear grandchildren, you have not been the forgotten ones. I continue to feel your loss and understand your pain. I pray that our Lord will guide you and keep you safe. May we as a family continue to find comfort in one another to help in our healing process, so that one day we all will find peace within ourselves.

To Gary Moss, our attorney, for your endless work, patience and understanding. You were committed to and fought hard to see justice done.

To Robert Reed, thank you so very much. You're a wonderful caring man who helped me coordinate this project which significantly impacted this book and consequently, changed my life.

Thank you, thank you, Colin Ingram and Jeanette Hartage. You started with a not-too-ordered lump of information and turned it into a book. Everyone should have editors like you, who leave me with no horror stories to tell.

To Paul Gigliello, Sr., for your continuing love and support for your son Paul, and to Diane, Paul's step-mom, we thank you.

To my siblings and their wives, Stephen and Karen, Lou and Catherine, Nick and Dolly, for your unconditional love and support during my time of need.

To Terri Keith, thank you for reaching out to us, and sharing your own painful experience. Your friendship has been so uplifting during some very hard times. Your strong convictions for change have been enlightening. It's a tough fight, but together we can win.

To Lucinda von Reichon, our adopted publicist, your support and dedication has been admirable. Because of your heroic effort in wanting to help people, you have made a difference. Thank you for your ongoing help and guidance in making our book a reality.

A special thank you to Grace Vessel ("Amazing Grace") for the spiritual gift you bestowed on us.

Contents

x

Foreword

As her sisters and brother stood sobbing, my mind flashed back to a time when the children were little. I was six months pregnant with Jenny. My husband, Lou, and I were getting ready to take the children to a show. It was a chilly, San Francisco winter night, and the heater was on to take the chill out of the house.

Suddenly, there were screams in the hallway. "Oh, my God, something has happened to the children," was my first thought. I was afraid of what I might find, as I grabbed my pregnant belly and ran to see what was wrong.

There, sitting in front of our wall heater, was a small bird. It had somehow flown into the house. I took a deep breath, feeling great relief that nothing had happened to the children. They were just startled and it was nothing a few hugs couldn't take care of.

After releasing the bird to safety outside, the evening passed as planned. An old wives' tale briefly crossed my mind. The tale says that when a bird enters your house, someone is going to die. I associated this with the bird, but never spoke of it to anyone and quickly dismissed the thought.

A few months went by, and I gave birth to a beautiful baby girl, Jenny. I remember counting all her fingers and toes, making sure my little girl was okay. She was perfect in every way. It wasn't until I brought her home from the hospital that I noticed the birthmark below her tummy. I was shocked. Not to find a birthmark, but to see that it was in the shape of a bird! For an instant I allowed that old wives' tale to enter my mind again, and I quietly asked myself if the life of this beautiful child would some day be taken from me.

I banished the thought until this day, as I stand over her life-less body. Now, 30 years later, my daughter is dead. There have been many questions for which we have no answers, but I can tell you with great conviction that I know my child did not die because of an old wives' tale or because a bird flew into our house.

Jenny died because of medical neglect, as that little bird would have died so many years ago had we not cared enough to help it out of our home and into a safer place. The truth is that her doctors just did not care.

The crying has stopped, our love never will.

Introduction

When my newlywed daughter, Jennifer Lynn Gigliello, proudly told me she was pregnant, I shared her excitement and happiness. I couldn't help but think back to the childhood days of this baby of the family, who, with her curly brown hair and infectious smile, danced and sang to entertain her family, her blue-green eyes sparkling. Now, a happily married 21-year old, she was seeing a dream come true (the dream of starting her own family). With eagerness and energy, she took me along, a willing partner, on weekly shopping trips for baby clothes. Vivacious and healthy, Jenny had no intention of slowing down.

Before her baby was born, though, Jenny experienced the first of many attacks of severe abdominal pain. These episodes continued, intensified, and came with increasing frequency for eight years (eight years of treatments, surgeries, and neglect that failed to correctly diagnose or resolve her illness). Each time she saw a new doctor, Jenny was convinced her problems would soon come to an end, and before long she could resume her normal activities. Finally, however, doctor and emergency room visits and hospital stays literally consumed her life, as she battled excruciating pain day after day. Her trust in doctors continued even after she came under the care of a health maintenance organization (HMO).

The neglect of one of the nations largest HMOs was the direct cause of Jenny's painful (and unnecessary) death. How many other patients have been maimed, crippled, or killed by similar treatment? How many more will suffer the same fate? How will you or someone you love be treated if your health insurer is an HMO? Records confirm that many patients receive inadequate care. Lawsuits against HMOs continue to be lodged, as families attempt to obtain fair and compassionate treatment from these organizations or to receive compensation for wrongful deaths.

A 1994 *New York Times* article by Bob Herbert accurately portrayed the system that killed Jenny:

> There is a new world of medicine in the United States, a world that pulsates to the impersonal and incessantly driving rhythms of corporate greed. Patients are not important in this world. They are little more than data entries in elaborate schemes to cut costs and bolster profits as radically as possible. The smart set calls it managed care. The corporate types love it. They have plunged into all phases of the health care system with their single-minded pursuit of financial gain, often at the expense of patients and over the concerns of caregivers....
>
> Managed care is, in essence, corporate care. Decisions that once were made by doctors are being taken over by executives obsessed with the bottom line. In that environment, patients can be processed as impersonally as any other commodity.

The results of this mindless worship of cost-cutting and corporate greed can be catastrophic. Second opinions or specialist care may be denied at the whim of an administrator. Patients or their families may be asked to perform tasks at home that are far beyond their knowledge or skills and that require close medical supervision. In addition, the maximum financial liability in California for wrongful death cases is $250,000, far less than the cost of caring for high-risk patients; this can lead only to the frightening conclusion that it is more cost effective to let some patients die than to treat them.

Massive amounts of propaganda are published by HMOs in order to gain new clients. Their attractive, full-color brochures tout highly skilled and compassionate care. But their big draw is lower insurance premiums and elimination of the burden of filing claims for payment of bills. Unfortunately, their definition of what is needed and when it is needed does not always coincide with the actual needs of the patient. Consumers need to be aware of the unique dangers they may face if they elect to have an HMO as their health care provider.

Throughout Jenny's illness, the different parts of the American health care system failed to communicate and work together in her best interest. Due to circumstances of employment, Jenny was covered first by private health insurance, then by MediCal (California's version of Medicaid), and finally by an HMO. Many of those involved in her medical care share some responsibility for her premature and needless death. The blame cannot be placed on any one individual. In some cases, the cause was lack of training; in others, inattention to detail; still others were too busy, perhaps overworked, or were overwhelmed with paper work. In some cases, necessary skills were simply not there, and one can't help but wonder whether some cared at all. The sad truth is that the day our Jenny died she still suffered from the same agonizing pain she first experienced eight years earlier.

The story you are about to read is as accurate in every detail as our family has been able to make it. We feel strongly that there are important lessons to be learned from our experience: lessons about choosing an HMO or an individual physician, about demanding the services of a specialist when no progress in the patient's condition can be seen within a reasonable amount of time; lessons about the necessity of having a vigilant patient advocate demanding proper care; lessons about seeking second and even third opinions; lessons concerning both the patient's and the family's need to become educated about the specific symptoms, illness, or procedures they face.

This book documents shocking neglect and incompetence by a major HMO. It also raises questions about certain protocols and practices: How can HMOs defend the dangerous pattern of failure to seek a specialist's intervention in difficult cases? Why are patients sent home from the hospital without adequate monitoring and training for complicated treatments? Do HMOs deliberately neglect and mismanage their difficult patients? It is, after all, cheaper to let them die. Why are medical records missing at critical times, when a patient's life hangs in the balance? What are they doing to ensure that the patient and a grieving family are treated with dignity, compassion, and respect? In our own case, when Jenny died she was left at the side of the bed like a rag doll, blood trickling from her mouth. None of those present expressed sympathy. They went about other tasks as if we didn't exist.

When Jenny had her first attack of pain, none of us dreamed that it was the beginning of the end of her life. It is still hard to comprehend all the suffering she endured in the years that followed. I do not include the sometimes gruesome details of Jenny's treatment to gain sympathy. Rather, I believe the story of our family's fifteen-year medical and legal nightmare can help change the way the American system of health care operates. If it doesn't change, what happened to Jenny and our family could just as easily happen to you and yours.

Dorothy Rose Cancilla
September 1, 1999
Rohnert Park, California

1

We Should Have Named Her Joy

A thing of beauty is a joy for ever:
Its loveliness increases; it will never
Pass into nothingness; but still keep
A bower quiet for us, and a sleep
Full of sweet dreams, and health, and quiet beauty.
John Keats

Family

Three-year-old Jenny laughed as she sang and danced for her family. She entertained us, her blue-green eyes sparkling and her brown curls bouncing. I often thought we should have named her "Joy" because she brought so much joy to us all.

I remember when Lou and I brought Jenny home from the hospital; the three other children stayed home from school so they could be there to greet their new baby sister. Right from the start they were thrilled and excited. Throughout the years our children shared a special bond, and nothing could ever come between them.

Our middle children, seven-year-old twins Cathy and Vince, wanted me to bring Jenny to their second-grade classroom so their teacher and the other children could see her. The teacher asked me to stand at the head of the classroom while the children all formed a line to come up and meet Jenny. I was touched to see Vince and Cathy stand patiently in line to see their own sister. They looked at her with the same awe as the other children, who had never seen her.

I didn't want to leave Jenny with babysitters, so I opened a small fur and gift shop on 24th Street in San Francisco. We lived over the shop. The other three children were attending St. Peter's Catholic School, about a block away, so for us it was the perfect solution.

As a little girl, Jenny was cuddly, outgoing, and adorable. Because she was the youngest member of the family, the three older children always fussed over her. The older ones had the usual disagreements and fights, but they never fought with Jenny. She was the baby of the family. She was special.

We went to the movies as often as we could afford it. One day the older children wanted to see Charlton Heston in "The Ten Commandments." Jenny was four years old and full of energy. She spent the first half of the movie running up and down the aisles of the theater. Because I couldn't get her to calm down, I finally told the manager we were leaving. He gave a sigh of relief, thanked me, and gave me two free passes for the next night.

Although she was the darling of the family, Jenny never acted like a spoiled child. In fact, it was Jenny who always tried to take care of everyone else. From an early age, it was clear that she put the needs of others before her own.

At Epiphany, her Catholic grammar school, Jenny got along well with the other children and the teachers. She tried to help other children who had less than she did, or who came from troubled families. She was quick to sense the pain in another person's heart. She often invited friends to stay overnight.

Jenny may have been spoiled with attention from her family, but she was never selfish or self-centered. I remember her tenth birthday party. After it was over, she said, "Mom, you don't have to give me a big birthday party and invite all my friends any more. I'm getting too old for that now. I'd rather be with you and Dad and my brother and sisters and just have a cake." Although she was young, she managed to express her feelings very well and showed a caring for others beyond her years.

We had a close, affectionate family and loved doing things together. Lou's hobby was gambling on the horses at the San Mateo track. He really believed that some day he would strike it rich. Fortunately, in later years, he realized that would never happen. He often took all the kids with him to the racetrack, and they would have fun gathering up the losing tickets. Sometimes he kidded Rosemarie, our eldest daughter, saying she should become a jockey because she was so tiny. Rosemarie had many hopes and dreams (but becoming a jockey was never one of them).

Every Christmas the children looked forward to going to their Uncle Nick's Christmas tree lot. With all its lights they thought it was the most beautiful place in the world. Lou and I sat in Nick's trailer while the children ran through the lot and picked out our family tree, which their uncle presented to them as a gift. In later years, when Jenny's siblings reached their teenage years and lost interest in the tree hunt, Jenny and Lou continued the family tradition.

Jenny was very close to her sisters and her brother and remarkably like her father in personality, although she was somewhat easier going than he. As the years passed, she developed into a happy, healthy young lady who had many friends. Jenny would often tell Cathy and Vince personal things that a teenage girl would never tell her mother and father—things about her friends and her dates. She respected her older sister, almost as if Rosemarie were her mother. They were ten years apart in age, and Rosemarie took Jenny under her wing. She often bought Jenny gifts and took her places. When Rosemarie and Robert, her fiancé, were dating, Jenny was often their companion at the zoo or on trips to Disneyland.

Jenny and Paul

At Balboa High School in San Francisco, Jenny was a good student. She talked about becoming a social worker, because her ambition was to help people. However, conditions at Balboa deteriorated rapidly during her junior year. Violence was increasing, and the school was plagued with drugs. She did not return to complete her senior year because of these social problems. She attended cosmetology school, then worked as a beautician for some months. She enjoyed the field, but hadn't decided definitely on a career.

When she was eighteen, Jenny began work as a medical receptionist. She loved the job, because she was able to do what she did best, working with people who needed help. She learned to do a number of different tasks. She took patients' blood pressures, did typing and filing, and learned how to take electrocardiograms. She spent much of her spare time with Rosemarie, who lived 60 miles away in Novato.

When she was 19, Jenny met her future husband, Paul Gigliello, at a party. They dated for about two years and soon fell in love.

"She was dating a friend of mine," Paul recalls. "All the kids from the Excelsior district of San Francisco hung out together. We met at a friend's birthday party, and from then on we were always going someplace and doing something with our friends. Jenny liked to shoot pool, go dancing at nightclubs, and go bowling. She was naturally athletic; she loved camping, swimming, and waterskiing. One of my cousins had a powerboat, and we spent a whole day waterskiing one weekend at Lake Mendocino. Jenny loved being up on skis. That night we cooked out over an open campfire and roasted marshmallows. She laughed and giggled the whole weekend."

Jenny liked Paul right away. "He's Italian, and he's macho," she said. She called him "a real hunk," and she was in top form herself. Pictures taken in the spring of 1977 show her as an attractive, curly-haired, smiling young woman; she was slender and athletic-looking.

Paul treated Jenny well, and her father and I gave them our blessing. They were married at Epiphany Catholic Church on March 19, 1977, when Jenny was 21 and Paul was 24. Her father and I were very proud to see her married and shared her excitement about the happy and healthy life she looked forward to.

A beautiful bride, Jenny glowed as she walked down the isle wearing the same wedding gown that I wore the day I married her father 33 years earlier. Because Paul was so much taller than she, Jenny wore tall, sparkled platform shoes, which brought the top of her head up to Paul's shoulders. As the ceremony began, Lou cried softly. Tender emotions overcame my usually feisty, funny, talkative husband

I was an aspiring singer before Lou and I married. I sang in public at every opportunity, even garnering a spot on KYA radio's amateur hour in San Francisco. After our marriage, a singing career no longer interested me. I sang to my children instead. My husband and family were the most important things in my life. I sang in public for the last time at Paul and Jenny's wedding reception at Seven Hills Restaurant in San Francisco.

After I finished singing "It's A Sin To Tell A Lie," Lou had to get in his two-cents worth. He sang his favorite tune, "Pennies From Heaven." After the dancing at the reception, the bride and groom went for a ride on San Francisco's famous cable cars. It was a very romantic wedding.

Jenny was as happy as any young woman could be after she got married. She had carefully saved money while she was working before her marriage, and she used much of it to furnish their new home. She had a flair for decorating, and she turned their South San Francisco apartment into a pretty, cozy home. In no time at all, it seemed, she filled their home with flowers, a waterbed, a bar, a fish tank and furniture she and Paul chose. They loved to have other couples over, so she did everything she could to make their home comfortable for their friends.

Happy Parents

When Jenny learned she was pregnant, she couldn't have been happier. I was the first one she told. "Mom," she said with an ear-to-ear grin, "I'm pregnant. You're going to be a grand-mother!" She couldn't wait to go out and start buying baby clothes. From then on, the two of us went shopping every week. She had already picked out most of the baby's clothes before she was four months pregnant. She loved being a homemaker. All she wanted out of life was a good marriage, a warm home, and five children.

Jenny couldn't wait to become a mother, and she had an uneventful pregnancy except for one episode. In December 1977, when she was four months pregnant, Jenny called me one morning and said, "Oh, Mom, I had so much pain last night." The pain radiated from her front to her back, and I wondered if it might be a gallbladder attack. Violet Gigliello, her mother-in-law, was with her that night, and made her some tea to soothe the pain. Jenny evidently never told her gynecologist about the incident. Since the pain didn't recur during her pregnancy, Jenny wrote it off as a fluke. We had no way of knowing that this was a premonition of the dark days that would come later. She spent the rest of her pregnancy preparing her house for her new baby, enjoying married life and playing with her dog, Tasha.

On the night Paul was scheduled to take her to the hospital for a Caesarean delivery, she started going into labor. Paul and Jenny met with the doctor at the hospital, and I arrived shortly after they did. There she was, sitting on the hospital bed with a big belly, and no baby yet. I was worried (but as her mother, I considered that my job!). Paul was holding her hand. He was happy but a little nervous. The nurse came in and gave her a shot to relax her, and in a few hours it was all over

When Jenny gave birth to little Paulie on March 10, 1978, she was overwhelmed with emotion. I went to the nursery with Paul and her to see him for the first time after his birth. She cried with joy, she was so happy. Tears rolled down her face. She said, "Look. Isn't he beautiful! This is part of me and Paul." Then she turned to me and said, "Mom, thank you for being my mother. Now I know what it is to be a mother."

Paul was a proud papa, and he was just as thrilled as Jenny. The night before Jenny came home from the hospital, he took his brother-in-law, Vince, out to a favorite hangout for a drink (or three) to celebrate the birth of his son. Jenny didn't like the thought of him out celebrating without her, and told him so the next day!

After five days in the hospital, Jenny and Paulie came to stay at our house on Madrid Street in San Francisco for a few days. Paul went to work every day, which gave me a chance to enjoy my new grandson. All three of our daughters stayed with us when their children were born. It was a special time of bonding. Paul came every night after work to visit.

Jenny fell into the role of motherhood naturally. She was very careful, attentive, and protective with the new baby. She didn't even want me to hold him. She fed him, changed his diapers and was always looking for something cute to dress him in.

I remember a picture Jenny took of Paul with the baby. Paul was a big music fan and had a fancy stereo system. He sat in a chair with headphones on, cuddling Paulie, who was just a few weeks old. Paul wanted to listen to his jazz (but he didn't want to disturb the baby). He was very gentle with Paulie and took good care of him. He was always glad to sit with him when Jenny went shopping or came over to my house.

Jenny was also a fine mother to Dante and Vincent, her two stepsons from Paul's previous marriage. They spent part of their time with Jenny and Paul, and she and the two boys had a warm, close relationship. She showed no favoritism to her own son, but treated the three boys the same, lavishing them all with love. She played and laughed as much with one as with the others. Paulie recalls that she often took them swimming at a nearby pool. His best memories were the times his mom would take him to Chuck E Cheese's for pizza, crack jokes with him, horse around with him on the floor and pretend they were wrestling. There was nothing standoffish about Jenny. She was a hands-on mother to her children.

Jenny's two stepsons became close friends with the children of her sister, Cathy. Cathy and Jenny used to babysit for each other. Cathy loved to be with Jenny because she made her feel good with her upbeat attitude and her enthusiasm. Jenny seldom, if ever, got angry with anyone. She was happy with her life, and it showed in everything she did. She wasn't a pushover, though. If she thought she was right, she held tight to her beliefs until someone proved her wrong. If that happened, though, she would accept the better idea and make it part of her life. She was tenacious, but open-minded, too, just like her father.

The first year of her marriage was the happiest time of her life. Marriage and motherhood were the culmination of Jenny's dreams. Everyone enjoyed her exuberance, and even her animals loved her. Tasha, her pet Pit Bull, slept at her feet, and her cockatiel, Bonkers, gave her a wolf whistle when she came into the room.

In April 1978, about six weeks after Paulie was born, Jenny had her second attack of severe abdominal pain, this time accompanied by vomiting of green bile. Like the first one she'd had during her pregnancy, the pain from this attack radiated from the left side of her abdomen to her back. Lou and I rushed her to a nearby hospital, where she was treated.

"We don't know what caused your pain," the doctor told Jenny when he dismissed her. Those words would haunt her for the next eight years. From then on, every time Jenny saw a new doctor, she was sure he would be the one to diagnose and treat her problem. She trusted her doctors to cure her. They didn't. Looking back, I am glad she had such a happy life when she was first married, because the years ahead were to become a long, agonizing, medical nightmare.

2

The Pain

*For all the happiness mankind can gain
Is not in pleasure, but in rest from pain.*
                                John Dryden, ca. 1675

Luck and Pancreatitis

Paul played poker with his buddies every week. One night
the game was dealer's choice, and the pots were substantial. Paul
was close to losing his entire paycheck.

"Let me play," begged Jenny. "I just got paid. Give me a
chance."

"Sorry," Paul said. "This is a man's game." She persisted,
though, and the men agreed to let her sit in for a while. In two
hours, she had won all Paul's money back.

"Hey Paul," the guys said, "next time, you stay home and let
Jenny play." From that night on, Jenny was a regular member of
the poker group. She also liked to go to the racetrack and place
a bet now and then, awakening memories of trips to the track
with her father when she was growing up. One weekend, when
she and Paul attended a wedding in Las Vegas, they each took a
hundred dollars to gamble with. Paul's stake was gone in an hour

(but Jenny came home with eight hundred dollars winnings in her purse).

Unfortunately, her luck didn't hold out where her health was concerned.

Jenny didn't have another pain attack for seven months. Then, just as before, she had strong pain in her abdomen, accompanied by vomiting. At the time, Paul and Jenny were both working for the Coen Company, a manufacturer of combustion burners. Paul did warehouse and assembly work there and Jenny worked in the office. Jenny was doing clerical work when the pain hit. She doubled up in agony, and vomited green bile. A supervisor called Paul, who was working in the shop. Paul took her to see her physician, Dr. Barbara Thomas, who admitted her to Mt. Hope Hospital. During the four hours she was there, the staff took x-rays, ran blood tests, gave her medications to relax her and take away the pain, and sent her home.

Dr. Alfred Ellis, Jr., a gastroenterologist at Mt. Hope, believed Jenny's problem was inflammation of the gallbladder or gallstones, and he recommended that her gallbladder be removed.

The gallbladder is a small sac about three inches long, located on the underside of the liver just below the lower ribs. Its function is to store bile secreted by the liver until it is needed in the digestive process. In normal operation, the gallbladder releases the bile into the biliary (bile) ducts and into the duodenum to aid digestion. If gallstones form in the gallbladder, the passage of bile can be partially or completely blocked. This blockage results in extreme pain, which is often centered in the lower right quadrant of the chest. Small stones are often expelled into the bile duct and may pass through the body without incident, but is also possible for gallstones to lodge in the pancreas. This can cause an irritation or inflammation of the pancreas, called gallstone pancreatitis.

Lou believed in preventive medicine, but didn't believe in depending on doctors for every little thing. He and I both thought that Jenny, 22 at the time, was too young to need a gallbladder operation. When Dr. Ellis recommended surgery, I called a close friend, also a physician, for advice. He listened to what we had been told and suggested that we get a second surgical opinion. He recommended a colleague and close personal friend,

Dr. Eric R. David, who had a practice in San Francisco.

Dr. David examined Jenny and concluded that her pain was not the result of gallbladder disease. He felt that she had pancreatitis.

The pancreas is a gland, six to eight inches long, located just below and slightly behind the stomach. It produces two vital secretions: enzymes that aid digestion, and insulin, which controls the metabolism of sugar. The enzymes are delivered to the intestines through the pancreatic duct. Insulin is produced by small groups of specially modified cells in the pancreas. If these cells are surgically removed or fail to secrete sufficient amounts of insulin, diabetes (an excess of sugar in the blood) may result. If not carefully controlled with insulin, diabetes can lead to extreme thirst, weight loss, respiratory problems, kidney disease, loss of eyesight, diabetic coma, and death.

Pancreatitis is most commonly associated with gallstones, alcohol abuse, and certain medications. According to the National Institutes of Health, patients with pancreatitis may have one or several attacks. These painful attacks, which often include vomiting, last from one to several days and usually require hospitalization. Pain may be localized, or it may radiate to the back. Acute relapsing pancreatitis is usually caused by gallstones, but may also be caused by other less common factors, including abdominal trauma, cancer, pregnancy, or abdominal surgery.

Dr. David believed an excess of amylase, a pancreatic enzyme, caused the pain. When Jenny's amylase and white blood cell count went up, her pancreas became inflamed, and she had extreme pain. Then the inflammation would subside, and she'd feel better again for up to several months.

Jenny's symptoms closely matched those of pancreatitis, but what triggered the attacks? Was it her pregnancy? Or was it a gallstone? Her pain symptoms were consistent with a gallstone lodged in the pancreas. The gallbladder may have produced one or more stones which lodged in the bile duct, causing the pain. She was young, healthy, and didn't drink or take drugs. If the cause was pancreatitis, what had brought it on? There was no answer for us.

We didn't know whom to believe: Dr. Ellis, who favored a

diagnosis of gallbladder problems, or Dr. David, whose diagnosis was pancreatitis. The deciding factor came to be my friend's recommendation of Dr. David. From that point on, Dr. Eric David was the man who directed the course of Jenny's treatment. We now know what we didn't know then: that our choice of doctors would lead to a series of preventable disasters.

Jenny continued to suffer from recurring bouts of extreme pain and vomiting. When they occurred, emergency room physicians would give her the standard treatment for pancreatitis: hospitalize her, cut off her intake of solid food, put her on intravenous fluids, give her painkillers, let the attack wind down, and send her home. Then she would be all right for a while, until the next attack. Soon, she was having an attack (and a hospitalization) nearly every month. In addition, she required an operation unrelated to her usual pain; she had a tumor of her left parathyroid gland removed.

Frustration and Appendicitis

Jenny's case was frustrating for her doctors because in the beginning they couldn't visualize her problem on their diagnostic instruments. They knew that she was in a lot of pain, but nothing showed up on her x-rays. They would tell her, "Jenny, we can't see anything. We don't know what's causing your pain." It was a refrain she heard over and over again. After several of her visits to the emergency room, one of the doctors suggested that perhaps she had a low tolerance for pain. I can see why they might have thought that, but it wasn't true.

Despite the fact that everyone in the family knew that Jenny was not a whiner or a complainer, and because of the doctors' questioning, we started asking ourselves if Jenny's pain was as bad as she said it was. When the doctors questioned her pain level, Vince recalls saying to Jenny, "You know, maybe you *do* have a low tolerance for pain. Maybe you should try to deal with the pain at home instead of running the doctors every time." He wasn't the only one who had doubts back then. We know now that those doubts were groundless, but we didn't know it then. I can only imagine how bad it must have made Jenny feel to think that her family didn't fully believe the magnitude of her pain.

At some point the doctors noticed a small, dark spot on

Jenny's pancreas, when they reviewed her x-rays. It appeared to be a small stone. That made the doctors all the more convinced that the problem was her pancreas.

Regardless of her frequent pain attacks, Jenny was alert and living her life at full speed ahead. She hated having to go into the hospital because it took her away from her husband and her son. She wanted nothing more than to be with them.

Paulie and I often went shopping when Jenny ended up being hospitalized unexpectedly. We took her slippers, a night-gown, and sometimes a robe. I also bought her a charm necklace and, periodically, charms to add to it (charms that brought her a special message, such as "Something Special," "God Loves You," "#1 Mother," "90% Angel"). Each time Jenny opened a gift her eyes would sparkle. They were special moments for me, too, because I knew they brought a little sunshine into her life.

Photographs taken in March of 1979 at Paulie's first birthday party show Jenny as a radiant, happy, active young wife and mother with a big smile on her face. Her hair was long, and she had a frizzy perm. She wore bell-bottom jeans and a shirt tied at the waist. Other pictures captured her riding herd on a roomful of rambunctious young children as she guided them through a day filled with cake, ice cream and party games. She had set a festive, colorful table. Each of the children had a birthday cupcake with a candle in it, a hat, and party favors. She helped Paulie open his presents and appeared to have as much fun as he and the other children did.

On March 21, 1979, at the request of Dr. Alfred Ellis, Jenny underwent further testing at Memorial Hospital. There they performed an endoscopic retrograde pancreatogram (an x-ray of the pancreas) along with a computerized axial tomography (CAT) scan and ultrasound pictures. After reviewing the results and all of her present and previous x-rays, CAT scan and ultrasound exams, radiologists discovered a stone blocking her main pancreatic duct.

By May 1979, Jenny was back at Mt. Hope Hospital in San Francisco for one of her recurring pain attacks when yet another painful problem arose. In tears, Jenny called me from the hospital.

"Mom," she cried, "I have such pain! It's altogether different from the usual one, and I don't know what's causing it." Jenny requested that Dr. David be notified, but the hospital staff didn't want to call him.

Mothers know instinctively when their children are in real pain, and to me it was clear that Jenny's new pain was both real and different from her original problem. "Oh, God," I prayed, "please, not another thing happening when she's already in such pain."

I called Dr. David and asked him to visit Jenny in the hospital. I said that it sounded like her appendix, but he initially said, "No, it sounds like more of the same pain she's in there now for." "That's not true," I insisted. "This pain is centered in her lower right abdomen, not her chest or back, as with the original pain." I finally convinced him to examine her again. As soon as he did so, he found that her appendix was severely inflamed and ready to burst. Dr. David performed an emergency appendectomy the same day.

That gave us some idea of just how much pain Jenny must have been going through, but Dr. David and the nurses initially wouldn't pay any attention to her. They didn't perceive the level of her pain, even though she was telling them about it in detail. You would think that in a hospital they would be sensitive to that kind of information from a patient. That wasn't the way it worked, however. Jenny had to call me to intercede, because neither the doctor nor the hospital staff were doing anything about her pain. Maybe they were too busy. Or maybe they didn't care enough.

The appendectomy incident reinforced in my mind something I had always known; people usually have a good grasp of what is happening in their own bodies, and doctors and hospital staff often don't pay enough attention to what their patients are trying to tell them.

MediCal, Hickman, and TPN

When Paul was laid off from the Coen Company late in 1979, he lost the private medical insurance that paid for the special care Jenny was beginning to need on a recurring basis. Jenny was no longer able to hold a job because of the increasing frequency of her pain attacks. This meant that when the pain struck, Jenny was no longer able to go to a private family physician who knew all the fine points of her case. While she had private insurance, Jenny could go to her primary care physician, who knew her and all the details of her case and who knew what others involved in her care were doing. In addition, if the case warranted it, she could also be referred to a specialist.

The family's low income and Jenny's disability eventually qualified her for federal Medicare benefits and for the California Medicaid equivalent, MediCal, but they were no replacement for the private medical coverage they previously had. Paul and Jenny quickly learned the difference between being a patient with private health insurance and one without. They learned that if you have private insurance, access to medical care is not a problem, but if you are poor or out of work and have to depend on the state to take care of you, you are at the mercy of the system.

Now that she had no insurance, Jenny had to get her medical care at places that would settle for the small fee (about $11.00 at the time),the State of California was willing to pay for her visit as a MediCal patient. Usually, Jenny now had to seek treatment at crowded outpatient emergency rooms where they knew little about her condition and had little time to learn. Her status as a MediCal patient also virtually guaranteed that she would not be referred to a specialist in pancreatic disorders.

Typically, a different doctor treated Jenny each time she had an emergency room visit. This rapidly became one of her chief problems; there was nobody in overall charge of her care. In addition, due to the time it took for her medical records to be updated, one emergency room doctor often didn't know what the other had done the day before.

Jenny's recurring episodes of nausea, pain and vomiting continued, until by the spring of 1980, she suffered from severe weight loss and malnutrition. Dr. David recommended an operation on her pancreas. He told us little about the operation other than that it would, in his opinion, alleviate her pain. We didn't ask if he had done such operations before, and we never asked what complications might arise. We trusted him completely.

Jenny entered the hospital on March 13, 1980, and Dr. David performed a pancreaticojejunostomy (a duct drainage of the body and tail of the pancreas). The operation revealed that the main pancreatic duct was indeed obstructed, that there was a stone in the duct and that there was a cyst in the tail of the pancreas (the part that manufactures insulin).

After the operation, Jenny was in good spirits and made a good recovery. But just three months later, we were all shocked when she had another severe attack (exactly the same as before the surgery). She was diagnosed as having alkaline/bile gastritis and dumping syndrome. This meant that the food she ate irritated her stomach and intestines, and she threw it back up. Her body could no longer get nutrition through the normal digestion of her food. Another way to nourish her had to be found, or she might die of malnutrition.

Because of the problems she was having digesting solid food, doctors at Mt. Hope Hospital recommended that Jenny have a Hickman catheter inserted, so that she could receive most of her nourishment in that manner.

A catheter is a flexible tube that is inserted directly into a vein, artery, body cavity, or organ. The purpose of a Hickman catheter is to permit foods to be introduced directly into the body without first passing through the digestive system. In Jenny's case, the catheter was placed directly into the superior vena cava, the large vein that returns blood to the heart. Catheters are routinely used when the patient is in the hospital and can be monitored closely. Because this catheter passes through an open wound in the body, infection is always a possibility, and close monitoring of the catheter and its entry point is vital.

When someone has dumping syndrome, it is necessary to rebuild their strength through a form of intravenous feeding called TPN, which stands for Total Parenteral Nutrition. TPN is a method of feeding a patient exclusively by a route other than the stomach and intestines. As early as 1964, solutions consisting of purified amino acids and dextrose were designed to be placed directly into the bloodstream. Until the 1980s, TPN required hospitalization for periods of up to several weeks (a costly procedure).

By the time Jenny was having her problems, doctors had developed effective care strategies to assure that patients who had catheters would be protected from infections. Catheter sepsis (contamination of the catheter) is a major threat to the patient's life, since the catheter leads directly into the heart. If an infection starts at the catheter site, it is transmitted quickly to the heart, which then pumps the blood directly to the lungs. If this scenario happens, the situation can deteriorate rapidly into staphyloccal pneumonia, which can kill the patient within a few days.

3

Surgical Madness

I will follow that system or regimen which, according to my ability and judgment, I consider for the benefit of my patients, and abstain from whatever is deleterious and mischievous."

The Hippocratic Oath

The Whipple Procedure

"Oh God! Not again!" I prayed over and over, when late night phone calls came from Paul. He was letting us know they were on their way to the hospital and were bringing Paulie to stay with us. My heart would pound in agony. Even now, when I remember those times, I experience the feelings all over again.

The doorbell would ring and I could feel the butterflies in my stomach. Paul would be standing just outside the door holding baby Paulie, all bundled up and protected from the cold. I could see the car still running. I tried to get a glimpse of my daughter, waving to her and hoping she could see me. As the car drove away I could almost feel her pain. The nights were dark with the exception of a lit candle I placed in front of the Blessed Mother. It seemed to bring a light of hope.

The days were long, but we had to stay strong. Paulie need-ed us. I remember taking him for short walks to our church. I found comfort there, and prayed endlessly, hoping the Lord would hear. Paulie and I lit candles and placed them in front of St. Jude, our patron saint. He was known to help those in great need.

Paulie looked forward to the afternoons because that was when he was able to visit with his mom. When we arrived and walked into Jenny's hospital room, she glowed with love and happiness at the sight of her son. The feeling was mutual. Paulie climbed up on her bed with excitement, laughing with joy. It was heartwarming to see, and for me, it helped compensate for all those sleepless nights.

By the summer of 1980, Jenny had been under treatment for over two years, but her original pain persisted. An ultrasound examination in June seemed to indicate a slight enlargement of her pancreas but no other apparent problems. A CAT scan showed the calcification of the head of the pancreas, unchanged since it was detected in November 1978.

The scan, considered more accurate than ultrasound, did not show visible enlargement of the pancreas.

At this time, Dr. Eric David recommended an operation known as the Whipple procedure. We have no idea why he chose this course of action. We now know that it was a risky, rad-ical and very uncommon form of surgery for routine pancreatitis. In surgical reference books and medical journal articles, the pro-cedure is listed as "very extensive and high-risk," and is normal-ly only used when the patient's life is in danger from cancer of the pancreas. Indeed, a 1984 medical textbook stated that "many professionals question the justification of the Whipple procedure because of the high mortality rate." In Jenny's case, there was absolutely nothing to indicate that she had cancer of the pan-creas, and neither Dr. David nor anyone else ever so much as suggested the possibility.

The Whipple procedure, a "long, trying operation," as its originator, Dr. A. O. Whipple, described it, includes removal of part of the pancreas, a portion of the duodenum (the first part of the small intestine), the gallbladder, the bile duct, and sometimes part of the stomach. The stomach, the cut end of the pancreas

and the common bile duct are then surgically connected to the
jejunum (the second part of the small intestine).

At no time did Dr. David explain the Whipple procedure
to us or to Jenny. He told us only that it would probably solve
her problem. He didn't mention that between *5 and 30 percent
of patients die from the operation.* If he had told Jenny or the
family what he was going to do to her digestive tract or of the
high risk associated with the procedure, there is not a snow-
ball's chance in hell that Jenny would have agreed to the operation.

Before the surgery, Jenny was forced to be relocated to a
depressing convalescent hospital for an overnight stay. Why?
Because of a MediCal ruling that limits the time for hospital stays.
She was transported by minibus, still in much pain, to a facility
that smelled strongly of urine. It was a traumatic experience for
her, as well as for me. Jenny had to be sent away for one night
and brought back to the hospital the next day. This is another
example of how money plays such an important role in our medical care and the patient's well-being comes second.

Dr. David performed the Whipple procedure at St. Gabriel
Hospital on August 20, 1980. He found the head of the pancreas
fibrotic, enlarged, and chronically inflamed. Laboratory examination of the head of the pancreas determined that the main pancreatic duct was unnaturally small due to a congenital (birth)
defect, and that the duct contained a stone.

Removing the gallbladder is a standard part of the Whipple
operation, but for some unknown reason, Dr. David failed to
remove it. Since Jenny's pain had continued, there was also dis-
cussion about removing the tail of the pancreas. However, since
the tail is the part that produces insulin, Jenny was afraid of
becoming a diabetic. Dr. David reassured her that even if she
became a diabetic, she could control her diabetes with insulin
and still have a good life. In the final analysis, the doctor decided there was no good reason to remove the tail, and it also was
left intact.

Why did the doctor choose to perform this radical, risky
operation in the first place? We will never know, but we must
consider several motives. The first would have been totally
altruistic. Whether he was right or wrong, he may have

seriously thought that the Whipple procedure offered Jenny the best chance for relief from her distress. Other possible motives, however, include ignorance, medical opportunism, ego, and greed.

If there was a problem with the head and duct of the pancreas, a partial pancreatectomy (a relatively simple, straightforward removal of part of the pancreas) may have taken care of it. Because Dr. David was a general surgeon and not a specialist, he could not have had extensive experience performing the Whipple procedure.

After the operation, Jenny had a great deal of postoperative pain. In addition, the surgical site became severely infected. It was so bad that when she went to Dr. David's office, he used his finger to zip open the wound. Jenny told us that the pain was excruciating. He cleaned the wound and packed it with gauze. It was one more horrible thing for her to go through.

Jenny remained a dedicated optimist. Every time she was hospitalized, it strengthened her resolve to get better. She never felt or acted like a victim or martyr. She never complained or said, "Why me?" She was just looking for someone to help her get well so she could go home and take care of her son. She had complete faith in her doctors. She felt deep in her heart that one of them would make her well again.

When Jenny was in the hospital recovering from a pain attack, from malnutrition, or from an operation, she spent most of her time visiting other patients and cheering them up. She continued to put the needs of others before her own. Often, when she was hooked up to an intravenous medication dispenser, she would walk down to the visitor's waiting room and talk to the people there. Everybody knew her. She made friends with everyone.

We would go to visit Jenny and find her in a room with another patient who was in pain. There was one woman I particularly remember, who had cancer; her pain was so severe that she was on large doses of morphine. Jenny stayed with her a great deal of the time. She would get up and go talk to her, constantly trying to make her feel better. When the inevitable happened, and the woman died, her husband brought Jenny flowers. I'll never forget. He told her, "My wife died much easier, thanks to you."

For the rest of 1980, Jenny did reasonably well in coping with her pain, but the complications from surgery added more and more problems to her life. She was hospitalized a number of times that fall and winter for more episodes of the original pain. The diagnosis: pancreatitis in the remaining body and tail of the pancreas.

No Vacation from Pain

In February 1981, six months after the Whipple, Jenny and Paul took a vacation. Jenny had never met her father-in-law, Edward Gigliello, and he sent airline tickets so the two of them could visit him in New City, near Nyack, New York. He owned a pro shop in a bowling alley there. Jenny loved that vacation. She and Paul drove three-wheeled, all-terrain vehicles through the snow, and they enjoyed music and dancing at a friend's night-club. About the time their planned week was ending, Jenny's pain syndrome struck again and she landed in a hospital near Nyack for a week.

There she told the doctor that she had undergone a Whipple procedure, and he was shocked. He asked if she had cancer, and she, of course, said no. The doctor told Jenny then that usually a Whipple procedure is performed, especially on a young person, only if they have cancer. That was the first time Jenny or any of us learned how radical the Whipple procedure was.

"If I had known how extensive the surgery was, I would never have agreed to it," Jenny told us later. The Whipple had solved nothing, but it had vastly complicated and endangered her life.

When she left the hospital for home, she was happy because she was coming home to be with Paulie, who was having a birth-day. In fact, she called me and asked me to go out and buy a bicycle for him. Even though she had spent the second week of her vacation in the hospital, she didn't want her little boy to think that she had forgotten to buy a present for his birthday. I'll never forget that. She didn't talk about her week in pain in the hospi-tal. Instead, she bubbled on about the city, how beautiful it was, and how many interesting people she had met. Jenny refused to be preoccupied with her medical problems. She wanted to get on with life.

With the loss of most of her pancreas came the loss of the

enzyme pancrease, which helps the body break down and absorb fat. For this shortage, her doctors prescribed regular supplemental doses of pancrease.

She also developed bile gastritis with bilious vomiting again, so her intake of solid foods was restricted. When she did eat, bezoars would sometimes form. (Bezoars are balls of fiber and food that attach themselves to the intestinal tract.) She loved pineapple, for example, but pineapple is fibrous and readily caused bezoars. They, in turn, brought on her pain and vomiting attacks.

Because her bowel had been shortened, she couldn't eat very much food. She also developed dumping syndrome again. She simply couldn't absorb the necessary nutrients, as her food passed so quickly through her digestive tract. This syndrome also caused flushing, sweating, weakness, dizziness, and headaches.

It wasn't long before she became emaciated. She lost so much weight that you could see her bones through her skin.

We all tried to help her. We each had our own theories; we encouraged her to take vitamins, take her enzymes, and take proper care of herself. We talked to her frequently on the phone, trying to figure out what was wrong with her. We also tried to communicate with and work with the doctors, but it was hard. Very hard.

By fall 1981, Jenny had undergone a vast array of diagnostic procedures and a pancreas operation but still suffered recurring bouts of nausea, vomiting, diarrhea, abdominal pain and weight loss.

Even when she went to the hospital, Jenny tried to keep her spirits up. There were a few times when she became frustrated with having to return again and again to the hospital. Spending the Christmas holiday season away from her family in the hospital would sometimes dampen her spirits. She wasn't immune to depression, just resistant. She found her illness very frustrating.

Dr. Hobson

Sometime in 1981 or 1982 Jenny became acquainted with Dr. George L. Hobson, a gastroenterologist at St. Gabriel Hospital. Jenny had been referred to him by Dr. David, and Dr. Hobson took Jenny under his wing. Because of her recurring gastric problems, he started her once again on Total Parenteral Nutrition (TPN) via a Hickman catheter at St. Gabriel Hospital. Later the TPN was done on an outpatient basis at home. He saw that she was malnourished, and he wanted to rebuild her general health through nutrition. He also worked to minimize her chances of becoming addicted to painkillers.

Dr. Hobson seemed to be a very caring man, and Jenny put her total faith in him, as she had with each of her previous physicians. He was going to make her a test case, using before- and-after pictures of her success for a medical journal article on malnutrition.

One of the chief problems that patients with chronic or recurring pain experience is a gradual buildup of resistance to painkillers. After dozens and dozens of doses, the painkillers tend to lose their effect, and larger, more frequent doses become necessary. With this increase in resistance and the need for larger doses comes the risk of addiction to these powerful narcotic drugs. To complicate matters, some caregivers seem to confuse the need for frequent painkillers with a desire to obtain unnecessary drugs for their narcotic effect. Jenny and our family often had to deal with this problem.

We could see that the pain medication was a big problem because, by this time, Jenny was in almost constant pain. Dr. David said to my husband, "We don't know why she's in pain or how much pain she *has*. And, you know, she *is* taking a lot of pain medication."

Lou asked, "Why are you giving it to her if you don't think she's in pain?"

The doctor admitted, "Well, we don't *really* know another person's pain threshold."

When Jenny had attacks of her original symptoms, the basic painkiller dosage prescribed wasn't enough to cope with the attack. So she would go into the hospital and ask for additional painkillers. One day when she went to the emergency room at Memorial Hospital with vomiting and pain, one of the doctors looked at her and asked, "Well, are you here for your fix?"

Her problems made her a difficult patient to deal with, and the hospital often didn't know what to do with her. We knew that she was in pain and that her need for pain relief was legitimate, but when a new emergency room physician looked at her medication records, he might easily conclude that she was just another addict looking for a fix.

When Jenny was under Dr. Hobson's care, he, too, was concerned about the level of painkillers she was using. He had her evaluated by a psychologist, who concluded that her pain was quite real, not imagined. Nevertheless, though we knew that she would not ask for something she didn't need, even the family sometimes had a lingering doubt about her need for all those doses of narcotic painkillers. As with many other patients with painful, chronic illnesses, she did become addicted to the painkillers prescribed for her, but she never got high from them, and she did not abuse the dosage. She took what she was supposed to take, and she took it on time. Nevertheless, she often ran into medical professionals who treated her like an addict who simply used drugs by choice.

On April 1, 1983, Jenny underwent her fifth major operation: a Roux-en-Y gastrojejunostomy with biliary diversion (gastric bypass to divert bile away from the stomach). It did not relieve her symptoms. She continued to experience recurring episodes of abdominal pain and vomiting. By this time, Jenny had developed chronic dependence on Demerol, a strong narcotic painkiller, and suffered from chronic malnutrition.

As she became progressively more ill, it became more and more difficult for her to care for her son. When she was at home, she valiantly took care of him and did her household chores. As her condition progressed, hospitalizations made normal home life impossible.

Jenny's frequent hospitalizations had a strong effect on Paulie. Being separated so often from his mother made him feel very insecure. Perhaps in compensation, he developed extremely strong feelings for Lou and me; he came to stay with us. When Jenny was home from the hospital, she took him back home and cared for him herself. As the hospitalizations increased, the amount of time Paulie spent with us also increased. He became very close to Lou. They were pals and did everything together. Cathy's children were Paulie's age, and she frequently offered to take Paulie for afternoons or overnight stays so that Lou and I had time for our own personal needs. Paulie never wanted to leave our sight. Jenny's recurring hospitalizations made him fearful, and he evidently thought that if he was separated from us, he would lose us, too.

Lou did a lot for Jenny, doing grocery shopping for her and making sure her nutritional needs were met. He was frustrated that her doctors were not curing the illness that plagued her.

He didn't think they were doing enough to get to the root of her problems. He wrote letters to several doctors, trying to get better information on her condition and even joined the Planetree Health Resource Center in San Francisco in order to get more specific information on her condition. He never stopped supporting her and trying to find ways to help her get well.

In June, she started vomiting bright red blood, a cupful at a time, and Dr. David admitted her again to St. Gabriel. Jenny, now 27, was malnourished and in severe distress. The doctors could not discover the source of her bleeding. The evaluation noted that she was dependent on Demerol, "...which Dr. George Hobson has worked long and hard to try to ameliorate." It also stated that she was receiving TPN at home under the care of Dr. Hobson. It closed by noting, "She will be continued on Demerol, although attempts will be made to minimize her dose and maximize the time intervals." Again her symptoms were treated without identifying the source of her pain.

After another hospitalization in August 1983, we returned Paulie to Jenny's care at home. We were concerned that she was taking Demerol every two to four hours for pain, in addition to Pancrease tablets with every meal to aid her digestion, but she managed well and was glad to have her son with her again.

Later that month she had a two-day episode of sweatiness, abdominal pain and vomiting. Paul found her in her bathroom, passed out on the floor after a relatively large evening meal. Despite attempts at home care, Jenny had two similar episodes in rapid succession and was taken to the hospital. There they again fed her through a Hickman catheter until she was strong enough to go home. Her use of frequent high doses of Demerol continued to be prescribed.

In September 1983, Dr. Robert L. Wicks of St. Gabriel Hospital reviewed Jenny's case. He suggested that she seek a surgical consultation with Dr. David Hinshaw of Loma Linda Hospital in San Diego, who was developing an experimental pancreas transplant procedure. Lou wrote to him and obtained information, but since the operation was unproven, Jenny was afraid to try it.

Between hospitalizations, Jenny enjoyed life. She cared for her husband and son and took pleasure in visiting friends and relatives. She would be in the hospital for days, sometimes for weeks, but when she came out she tried to be as normal as possible. She didn't complain, and she never talked about her illness. There was nothing pathetic about Jenny.

4

The Hickman Wilderness

I will practice my profession with conscience and dignity. The health of my patient will be my first consideration.

The Declaration of Geneva,
World Medical Association, 1983

Family Reactions

"Finally, we're going to get to the bottom of this!" Each time Jenny was hospitalized this was her reaction. Then she was discharged and felt good for a while and was her usual, active self; but then there would be another episode of the same old problem. Doctors seemed at a loss to identify the source of her pain.

Each family member had a different reaction to Jenny's pain, hospitalizations and operations. Rosemarie and I nearly always went to the hospital and sat in the waiting room until we heard the news. When a procedure was over, Rosemarie would go to the phone and call Lou, who waited anxiously at home for news. When Rosemarie told him Jenny was okay, he would break down in tears of gratitude and joy.

Cathy didn't come to the hospital for several of the surgeries. "I had a hard time going to the hospital and seeing her sick. When I did, I felt anxious, like I was going to pass out. This made me feel guilty, because I wanted to be there and be supportive for my sister, but I couldn't. It was too hard."

"I felt so helpless when Jenny was in the hospital," Vince recalls. "It was hard to see her suffer. Just when things seemed to be going well, she would be right back in the hospital."

When he was living out of the area and couldn't visit, he would call Jenny and play music on the phone for her, hoping to cheer her up and take her mind off her pain. He felt relieved and temporarily comforted when Jenny laughed.

The increasing frequency of Jenny's pain attacks led to longer and more frequent periods of hospitalization. The amount of time she spent out of the hospitals was shrinking; the time spent as an inpatient was increasing. When Jenny was at home and in pain, she could not keep food in her stomach and frequently threw it back up. This led to malnutrition, and malnutrition led to hospitalization until her physical condition and stamina could be rebuilt.

In the fall of 1983 Jenny and Paul decided to move to Novato. They wanted to get away from the problems of urban San Francisco, live near Rosemarie, and raise their family in a place with a nicer climate. Although Jenny was often in and out of the hospital, she still believed that her problems would sometime end, and she wanted to raise her family in the country.

The move brought on a problem Jenny had not anticipated. When she got sick again, the first person she called was Dr. Hobson. The problem was that once she moved away from San Francisco, he was not able to treat her as his patient any more.

Dr. Hobson may have been as frustrated as Jenny with her lingering condition. He was well aware of the intensity of her pain. He was concerned that she was becoming addicted to the painkillers. However, he became annoyed with Jenny's long-distance, after-hours calls for help.

Situations like this are common with chronically ill patients, but Dr. Hobson was not prepared for them. Ultimately, his involvement with Jenny was limited by her decision to move to Novato.

When she was admitted to the hospital, she called Dr. Hobson, hoping for his advice and reassurance, but he told her he simply could not continue as her physician because of the distance. It was understandable enough, but Jenny felt betrayed. She was sick, she was in an emergency room in a new hospital where no one knew her medical history, and she felt abandoned. Jennifer really cared about Dr. Hobson. She thought he would be the answer to all her problems. Like all the other doctors before him, he wasn't.

Jenny continued to have to deal with those who treated her as a nuisance and an addict. One day she was hospitalized at Kaiser Permanente Hospital and her medical records said that she was to receive the painkiller Dilaudid every three to four hours. When her medication was late and Jenny asked for it, one of the nurses remarked, "Well, little Jenny is just going to have to wait today." Her tone made it clear that the nurse didn't think she was in any real pain.

Home TPN

Doctors at Kaiser often saw her determination as evidence that she was addicted to painkillers and was looking for a fix. It was a catch-22 for Jenny. The harder she tried to convince the doctors that her pain was real, the more she sounded like an addict looking to get high. With this kind of treatment from Kaiser, it didn't take long before Jenny became paranoid about going to them for the life-sustaining health care she desperately needed.

Hospitalizing Jenny and nourishing her by intravenous feeding in the hospital was time-consuming and expensive. In the 1980s, Home Parenteral Nutrition (HPN), a refinement of TPN, surfaced as an alternative to hospitalization for malnourished patients like Jenny.

However, to be safe and effective, candidates for HPN must be carefully trained before they start on this technically demanding form of nutritional therapy. In addition, the need for professional monitoring of the patient is even greater. To provide proper medical supervision, a trained nurse needs to visit the patient's home periodically, and a special TPN care team must supervise the program from the hospital. This was a tested method of treating malnutrition by the time it was used with Jenny.

This innovative system of home health care offered two potential benefits: a friendlier climate for the patient's recovery and much lower cost to the health care provider, since the necessity of extended hospital stays would be eliminated. It sounded great, but the lack of training and supervision that plagued Jenny's treatment was one of several fatally weak links in her care.

HPN, still commonly referred to as home TPN, depends upon two devices that work together to deliver fluids directly into the body. The first is a special pump; this delivers precise amounts of fluids into the bloodstream by way of a Hickman catheter.

The Hickman catheter is one of the more useful medical devices invented in this century. If not used and monitored properly, however, it is also one of the most dangerous. It consists of a long silicone tube about 1/8-inch in diameter. One end is inserted into the vena cava, as mentioned before; the other end has a cap that permits the introduction of liquids. The tube is held in place by a Dacron felt cuff. To insert the Hickman, two surgical incisions are required—one just above the collarbone, and the other to the side of one breast.

Jenny had a series of Hickman catheters implanted to deliver nutrition, painkillers, and later, insulin. Right from the start, the Hickman catheter implants created two new major health problems for Jenny: blood clots and infections.

Regular cleaning of the catheter, the site where it exits the body, and the dressing that keeps the site clean are essential to prevent clogging or contamination. The patient and health care workers assisting the patient must be specially trained and constantly alert for signs of infection at the exit site. In addition, the catheter, which is always full of blood, must be flushed every 12 hours with heparin to ensure that clotting does not take place and interfere with the proper flow of nutrition.

Dr. Molly Hackett of Memorial Hospital's Nutritional Support Service wrote that home TPN therapy was a well-accepted, safe method of treatment, but that it required comprehensive, daily monitoring by a physician and a nursing staff specifically trained in TPN therapy. A home TPN program must provide comprehensive patient education and instruction, and provide qualified

24-hour emergency nursing, pharmaceutical, and medical care. It must also conduct continuous home patient monitoring via visiting nurses and regularly evaluate all outpatient TPN patients in a hospital-based clinic. Every member of the home TPN staff must be able to recognize and treat TPN-related complications, such as catheter infections. And any hospital that fails to provide these services or has physicians who are incapable of diagnosing and treating TPN-related complications should not be administering home TPN therapy. If only someone had told us that in the early 1980s.

That October, Jenny's abdominal pain got worse. By then, she had moved to Novato. She was seen in the emergency room of North Bay Community Hospital where an abdominal x-ray showed distention of her bowels. They put a tube down her nose and drained off nearly two liters of fluid. As with most of her other problems, the cause of the gastric outlet obstruction was never determined. She was transferred to Memorial Hospital, where she was described as a "wasted, chronically ill-appearing young woman." There, Dr. Allen G. Stokes, a pancreas specialist, felt that use of a feeding tube directly to her stomach would "avoid pancreatic stimulation." A tube was placed through her nose; Dr. Stokes also surgically placed a feeding jejunostomy tube directly into her stomach. She tolerated the tubes fairly well and was discharged to recover at home. As usual, her recovery was short-lived. The next month she was again struck with pain, nausea and vomiting. This time she lost 22 pounds.

It was pouring rain when Rosemarie took Jenny back to Memorial Hospital in December. It seemed to her that every time she took Jenny to the hospital, it was a rainy day, usually a downpour, sometimes raining so hard that she would have to pull over to the side of the road. Extensive testing notwithstanding, the doctors reached no conclusion as to the cause of Jenny's symptoms. After ten days of treatment with three antibiotics, Jenny was released.

The 28th year of Jenny's life, 1984, started in pain, and her fifth Hickman catheter was inserted. Jenny also received training for home TPN, so that she could self-administer her nutritional fluids. In the hospital things seemed to go well, and she was discharged a week later. By the end of the month she was back to square one again. She was admitted to Memorial Hospital with sweats and chills from staph infection caused by the Hickman. That put her in the hospital for two weeks. While she was there, the doctors found that she was resistant to several common antibiotics, which had little effect on her infections. This was duly noted in her patient records. Jenny spent the rest of the year in and out of the hospital following severe bouts of abdominal pain, nausea, vomiting and weight loss.

A Botched Job

One might think that a chronically ill woman in constant pain who had a four-volume medical history would withdraw into a world of medicines and painkillers, but not Jenny. In 1984 she and Paul formed "It Takes Two," a household and apartment cleaning service in Novato. Even though she was ill and constantly in pain, she wanted to live a normal life and be self-sufficient. She made up fliers, advertised, answered the phone and developed a number of clients for her new business. "She wanted to do everything," Paul remembers. "Run a business, cook, clean house, take care of the kids. She didn't want to be treated like she was sick. She had more energy than I ever had. She was tough."

In February her Hickman catheter site again became infected and she was admitted to Memorial Hospital. Dr. Richard Norris wrote a detailed five-page report on Jenny's medical history. The frustration that the doctors were feeling over her case showed in the opening sentence. It read, "This is a 27 year old white female with an unfortunate medical and surgical course..."

After reviewing all the reports, Dr. Stokes felt that the remaining portion of Jenny's pancreas was the source of her recurring problems and recommended that it be removed. The family agreed.

On May 10, 1984, Jenny underwent her sixth major surgery. It was a pancreatectomy (a removal of the remaining part of her pancreas) performed by Dr. Allen G. Stokes. We were all worried, of course. When Rosemarie and I went into her room, we heard her mumble, "Look at all the unicorns." We knew that Jenny loved unicorns, and we thought it was a sign that she was having good thoughts. After all her miseries, we were desperate for a good sign. That's how we interpreted her unicorn dream:

a sign that everything was finally going to be okay.

Dr. Stokes noted that the pancreas "consisted of a small, extremely scarred and indurated remnant which was very abnormal looking. It was obvious that the patient suffered from advanced pancreatitis and that this could serve as the source for her pain." He also noted that the "small markedly diseased organ" had made diabetes a virtual certainty and that its removal would not increase that risk. The operation went well, and Jenny was returned to the recovery room in stable and good condition.

When the operation was over, Dr. Stokes came into the waiting room with a pained expression on his face. He was obviously holding something back. He said Jenny was doing all right, but there seemed to be something he wanted to say but couldn't. During the operation, Dr. Stokes had the opportunity to see how previous operations had been carried out. Some time later, an associate of his told something startling to a friend of Jenny's. The associate had heard Dr. Stokes comment that he'd never seen a surgery so badly botched as the Whipple operation performed on Jenny.

Now Jenny was diabetic, and every three or four hours she had to test her blood sugar level and take food if indicated. This left her even more dependent on medical technology, and gave her one more thing that could go wrong on short notice.

From the days of Jenny's first pain attacks, the family had always wondered if her gallbladder had something to do with her problems, even though we had gone with Dr. David's original diagnosis of pancreatitis and her June 1980 ultrasound examination at Mt. Hope Hospital had showed no gallbladder problems or gallstones.

Now, four years later, Dr. Stokes wrote to Dr. Henry Barber of Kaiser Permanente Medical Center, noting that "I am skeptical that the gallbladder has a major role in producing her symptoms... Nevertheless Jennifer has an unusual problem to say the least. I recommend that the gallbladder be removed and at the same time a feeding jejunostomy [tube] be inserted. Our previous experience demonstrated that she tolerated being nourished in this way, and it certainly would be easier and less expensive than intermittently hospitalizing her for total parenteral nutrition." The gallbladder was never removed.

The Catheter Time Line

Jenny had a well documented history of difficulty with her Hickman catheters. Between 1980 and 1986 she experienced several catheter related complications and had to have her catheter removed and replaced numerous times.

Jenny's first Hickman catheter had been implanted in June 1980, but multiple complications, including a pulmonary embolism (a blood clot in the artery between the lungs and the heart) and catheter infection forced removal of the catheter.

The second came in June 1982. It was left in place until she recovered sufficiently to take foods by mouth, and again the catheter was removed.

In September 1982, the third was placed. This catheter was removed after its insertion site became infected. The infection subsided after antibiotics were administered for ten days.

Jenny developed a pulmonary embolus after her fourth Hickman was implanted in March 1983. This resulted from flushing a clotted catheter; she was again admitted to St. Gabriel for pain, vomiting and inability to eat.

The fifth Hickman was placed in January 1984. It resulted in a recurring catheter infection that required a three-week stay in Memorial Hospital for intravenous antibiotic therapy. The physicians there spotted the infection right away, gave her antibiotics, determined which ones weren't working, noted this on her medical charts, and changed the antibiotics. They practiced good medicine. She recovered fully. You might say this was the bright spot in the Hickman wilderness.

Jenny's final Hickman catheter was placed in November 1985, after she had managed without one for over a year. Someone should have been watching closely for problems. Her history of recurring bouts with pulmonary embolisms and infections were a clear warning sign that something was wrong with the Hickman system. After the first problem, her physicians should have reviewed the techniques and procedures she used to care for and clean her catheter, in an attempt to prevent further complications. They should also have been prepared to start aggressive antibiotic therapy and/or remove the Hickman at the first sign of catheter infection.

At the age of 28, Jenny had been in pain for seven years with little relief. She had been through six major operations, including a major resection of her bowels, had her pancreas removed, was diabetic, and dependent on narcotic painkillers.

Still she had the identical problems of seven years before (severe recurrent abdominal pain and vomiting). We tried to hide our feelings from Jenny, but we were getting frantic.

5

The Kaiser Experiment

Being a good doctor means being incredibly compul-
sive. It has nothing to do with flights of intuition or bril-
liant diagnoses or even saving lives. It's dealing with a lot
of people with chronic diseases that you can't really
change or improve.... You can make a difference in their
lives, but you do that mostly by drudgery (day after day
paying attention to details... and being responsive on the
phone when you don't feel like being responsive).

John Pekkanen, M.D.,
Doctors Talk About Themselves

Kaiser Beginnings

I was delighted when Jenny and Paul moved to Novato, in
Marin County, in the fall of 1983. The move had given Paul the
opportunity to take a job with the S. T. Johnson Company, another boiler-making firm. They offered health insurance as one of
their fringe benefits, and soon he and Jenny were registered with
one of America's largest health maintenance organizations: Kaiser
Permanente Medical Center.

Kaiser Foundation Health Plan of Northern California was a

force to be reckoned with in the health care field. By 1995 they were the primary care providers for nearly 2.5 million residents of northern California. This Kaiser plan alone employed over 3,366 physicians and operated 16 hospitals and 32 medical office buildings.

Jenny was immediately impressed with Dr. Henry Barber, her primary care physician at Kaiser. His specialty was internal medicine and gastroenterology. Now she finally had private health insurance again. She respected Dr. Barber. She felt safe.

The remainder of 1984 and 1985, though, continued to play out in what had become a mind-and-body-numbing routine for Jenny. By 1984 she was never out of pain. Sometimes it got the best of her; sometimes it didn't. In 1985 the doctors increased the strength of the pain medication she was taking intravenously through the Hickman catheter. From that point on, she took Dilaudid on a continuous basis, and she was drug dependent. The constant pain was so great that she couldn't get through the day without it (but she still tried to lead a normal life).

Previously she had taken her painkillers by injection into the muscles of her arms and legs. Paul recalls that by the time Kaiser started her on home TPN, that was no longer possible. "Every time I'd give her a shot, the medicine would squirt back in my face. She had no more muscles left."

This led to Kaiser instructing her to inject the painkillers directly into the Hickman catheter, a role never envisioned to be a part of home TPN. This required regular flushing of the catheter line, a demanding technical procedure previously performed only by trained technicians. "That was way over my head," Paul stated. "It was way over Jenny's head, too."

The problem was compounded by Jenny's need to inject insulin to control her blood sugar level. Kaiser had her inject the insulin into the Hickman catheter. "Kaiser never told us that home TPN would be so complicated," Paul recalls. "They made it sound as though she'd hook the Hickman up to the pump overnight, unhook in the morning, and walk around free as a bird. They told her that if she felt dizzy from her blood sugar dropping, to just suck on a lollipop. In fact, the home TPN program was a nightmare.

"Every time she had to inject medicine, she'd have to clamp

the Hickman line, stop the pump, inject the medicine, flush the line, unclamp it, and restart the machine. She had to do this at least every three hours during the day."

Page after page in my notebook is filled with records of Jenny's trips to the hospital. The doctors kept treating the symptoms, but never got to the root of her problem. Time after time she was readmitted to the hospital for the exact same problem. This is the kind of life she had in 1984:

May 26, 1984. Admitted to Kaiser for chronic abdominal pain; discharged May 29.

June 12, 1984. Admitted to Kaiser for dehydration, abdominal pain, vomiting and nausea. Discharged June 15.

June 16–July 27, 1984. Admitted to Kaiser for pain and vomiting and what was thought to be a small bowel obstruction. None was found.

August 7–11, 1984. Readmitted to Kaiser after having developed a grand mal seizure.

September 9–17, 1984. Readmitted to Kaiser.

September 27–October 1, 1984. Readmitted to Kaiser.

October 2–7, 1984. Readmitted to Kaiser.

October 9–11, 1984. Readmitted to Kaiser.

October 16–23. Readmitted to Kaiser.

After additional problems with her Hickman catheter, and on the recommendation of Dr. Allen Stokes, Jenny had a feeding tube surgically inserted into her digestive tract in December 1984. "This procedure was not successful," Dr. Stokes wrote. "The site became badly infected and the tube was removed a short time later."

Outrage and Optimism

Paul recalls just how badly infected the feeding tube was. "When I was visiting Jenny in the hospital, she complained that the feeding tube site was raw and sore. They were using the tube regularly to feed her, and it hurt a great deal each time they hooked her up. The outside of the tube, which went through her abdominal wall and into her intestine, was wrapped with gauze bandages. When I pulled down the covers and lifted the edge of the bandage I saw yellow-green pus oozing from the site. The dressing itself was half hanging off. They were supposed to change the sterile dressing every day and be alert for infections, but they weren't.

"I called a nurse. She said, 'Well, we have to see if the feeding tube is going to work or not.'

"I was outraged. I replied, 'What are you talking about? Any fool can see that this thing is badly infected. Look at the pain my wife is in. Look at the round red circle of inflammation around the tube. Look at the pus coming from the wound. It's not going to get uninfected by itself.' They pulled the tube a short time later that day, but only because I (Jenny's medically untrained husband) found the problem, not the doctors or nurses. That's the kind of care Jenny got."

By the next spring, all her usual problems were still afflicting her. Another feeding tube was inserted in April, but it, too, led to infection and was removed. Before the end of the summer of 1985, Jenny was hospitalized five more times for the same symptoms: vomiting, abdominal pain, malnutrition and dehydration. Each time they kept her in the hospital for four or five days until her condition stabilized, and then sent her home until it happened again the next month.

Despite all the pain, vomiting, medications, machines and tubes, Jenny kept trying to lead a normal life. One of my most precious mementos is a videotape we have of her at Rose's 40th birthday party in July 1985. Jenny was in high spirits, up and about and dancing with all the members of the family to tunes like "Jailhouse Rock," "Shake, Rattle, and Roll," and "Beer Barrel Polka."

That brief interlude of pleasure changed nothing, however, and in August she was back in Kaiser Hospital for all the old problems. Jenny spent the rest of 1985 the same way she started it (in and out of the hospital every few weeks, and always with the same horrible problems).

Prior to her last operation, which left her an insulin-dependent diabetic, Jenny had been able to bounce back fairly quickly from her bouts of malnutrition. With diabetes added to her already considerable list of problems, she no longer recovered as quickly as before. Nevertheless she kept a positive mental attitude and fought whatever problems she was experiencing. She monitored her own blood sugar levels, she injected her own insulin, she calibrated and ran the TPN pump, and she cleansed the Hickman line. She never complained, and she held to the belief that everything that happened to her was a temporary set-back from which she would recover. Jenny still found it hard to accept the fact that she was sick. Unlucky? Perhaps. Sick? No. She continued to be a happy, active person who wanted to be a good mother to her family.

Perhaps because of her unflagging optimism, we came to accept all the hospital visits and crises as a normal way of life. Until the last weeks, none of us saw her problems as truly life-threatening. We had taken her to the hospital so many times that one more time was no longer a big deal. We took her in, they fixed her up, we took her home. We, too, thought of the admissions as temporary setbacks. We had become accustomed to them.

In the middle of November 1985, Jenny had an extremely bad bout with pain and malnutrition. She was hospitalized at Kaiser for six weeks to build up her general health. She was in the hospital during both Thanksgiving and Christmas, and wasn't discharged until the middle of January 1986. Spending Christmas in the hospital was very depressing for her. She spent a lot of time crying.

Jenny, the Pro (Kaiser, the Amateur)

From the start, the Kaiser staff repeatedly demonstrated that they knew practically nothing about TPN or how to administer the TPN nutrients and medications by way of the dosage pump and the Hickman catheter. Jenny had to instruct the Kaiser staff on how to calibrate and use the pump that regulates the dosage of drugs and nutritional supplements into the Hickman catheter. When she was hospitalized at Kaiser, the nurses would often reach to start the pump before Jenny was ready or before the pump had been properly calibrated. Jenny would have to stop them and tell them what was wrong. They didn't know what to look for by themselves.

They were also unaware of the proper sterile procedures for changing the needles on the intravenous tube that feeds into the Hickman catheter. Besides that, they didn't know the proper procedures for keeping the site clean where the Hickman passes through the chest wall. One day, Kaiser's Dr. Barber chewed out the nursing staff for not using sterile procedures and not having changed the sterile dressing on the Hickman entry site on her chest. This kind of negligence and ignorance was a real menace to her health. If proper sterile procedures weren't followed, Jenny could become seriously infected through the Hickman or at the point where the Hickman line passed through the chest wall.

At home, Jenny used the TPN pump all night. The pump administered 3,000 ccs (about three quarts) of hyperalimentation nutritional fluids and medications. The medications included Dilaudid, a painkiller, and Valium, a tranquilizer. She had a complicated procedure to perform every night when she hooked up to the TPN pump. First she had to sterilize her hands by washing them in alcohol. Next she would sterilize the line with alcohol and Betadine solution. Then she would connect the tube to the TPN pump. She also had to flush the line with saline solutions and heparin, a blood thinner, to keep the line from clogging. It was a complicated procedure, and prone to infection. She had to flush the line every two or four hours when she took the Dilaudid.

During the day the pump would be turned off, the needle from the TPN supply removed from the Hickman, and she would tape the external part of the Hickman line to her chest and try to live a normal life. The problem was that TPN didn't solve all her nutritional needs. After varying periods of time, she would become malnourished again and land back in the hospital.

Jenny was the first TPN patient that Kaiser Hospital of San Rafael tried treating at home as an outpatient. They said that home treatment was better for her. In fact, their chief motive for prescribing home TPN for Jenny was financial; having her out of the hospital saved them money. The staff at Kaiser had never before managed the care of a TPN patient at home, but they were going to try with Jenny. She was their experiment.

We knew that home TPN required a staff of caregivers who were specially educated in TPN and the use and care of the Hickman catheter. Proper care also required that a protocol (a rigid set of standards) be developed and used. It also required the vigilant oversight of a trained group of medical supervisors who were supposed to monitor caregivers and be alert for any sign of problems, especially infections. At Kaiser, we later learned, none of these criteria were met.

After her hospitalization in the winter of 1985-86, Kaiser supposedly introduced a new protocol covering Jenny's home care. The protocol was useless, for none of the caregivers knew how to use the equipment or keep the system sterile. Jenny knew more about the system than all of them. One day Jenny called me from the hospital. She was all excited. "Mom, one of the nursing supervisors said I'm so good at taking care of myself that they want me to come back and teach the nurses how to use the equipment," she said. Jenny took it as a great compliment. What it showed, however, was an appalling lack of knowledge on the part of the people entrusted with her life.

Two weeks after she went home, she was back at the Kaiser emergency room with pain and vomiting. Nothing had changed.

At some point during Jenny's first months with Kaiser, the staff stopped viewing Jenny as a patient to be healed and started treating her like a problem they wished would go away. Dr. Barber, the man in charge of her care, worked with her often, but when he was away, the staff made it clear in myriad ways that Jenny was a nuisance they'd rather not deal with. We learned that none of the internal medicine physicians but Dr. Barber wanted to have anything to do with Jenny.

Neglect and Reality

Dr. Barber compounded the problems by failing to make the necessary special notations about Jenny's care in her medical charts when he left for conference or on vacation. The consequences were severe. On one occasion Jenny went to the emergency room in a malnourished state. She weighed only 75 or 80 pounds, and instead of giving her nutrients, they gave her only an intravenous drip of glucose. When she went in with severe pain, they would withhold the painkiller, thinking that she was there for a fix.

Paul recalls one night when Jenny called him from the hospital in severe pain. Dr. Barber wasn't around. In tears, she told Paul, "They're giving me water and placebos. They won't give me my pain medications. I hurt so bad. Please call somebody."

"Even after treating her for many months and many visits, they would pull stunts like that to see if she was really in pain or just there to get a fix. Kaiser treated her like a laboratory rat. It was inhuman," Paul complained.

Even though Jenny and Paul asked Dr. Barber to leave special instructions in her charts if he was going to be out of town, he failed to do so, and Jenny suffered needlessly.

The last two years before her death, our family never grasped how serious her condition was. Maybe we didn't know; maybe we didn't want to know. Or maybe we knew and we kept ourselves in a state of denial. I don't think we'll ever know for certain.

I kept hoping that her pain and vomiting was being caused by the large doses of drugs she was getting every day. When you are on painkillers, your system reacts abnormally, and I hoped that Jenny's delirious episodes were just from the drugs. Yet inside, I was angry, very angry, at the doctors who took her in and sent her home without ever figuring out what was wrong with her.

Paul's frustration continued at the way they treated Jenny. Once while he was with her in the hospital, a staff member seemed to be accusing her of coming in to get a "fix" of morphine for the high she would get from it. Paul almost punched him out on the spot. Sitting at home in their refrigerator was a huge bottle of morphine (enough for at least 150 doses) which the hospital provided for her normal daily use.

I was angry, too, at the harassment Jenny received at Kaiser. They would admit her, put her on intravenous medications and supplemental feeding, and tell her not to eat anything. Jenny was severely malnourished, and they told her not to eat! Once she became rebellious and asked Paul to bring her a turkey sandwich. Jenny knew that if she ate it she would probably have problems digesting it, but she was so starved for normal food that she had the sandwich smuggled in anyway.

She sneaked into the bathroom to eat it; but the nurse stormed into her room, pounded on the bathroom door, and accused this malnourished, starving young woman of going into the bathroom to use illegal drugs!

Her long-term illness had another effect on us. We started to wonder if part of it was Jenny's own fault. There were times when I got mad at her because I thought that maybe she wasn't taking good care of herself. That wasn't true, and I felt guilty about even thinking that. But long-term illnesses are hard on the people around the patient, as well as on the patient. With Kaiser's doctors constantly inferring that Jenny was part of her own problem, it made it inevitable that we would suspect our daughter of neglecting herself. It wasn't true, but that's the kind of nagging doubts we had sometimes. When someone has a chronic condition, you don't know what or who to believe, because nobody can do anything about it.

One of the hardest things for Jenny to accept was the realization that she probably would never be able to have more children. This pain was as real as her physical pain, because her family was her life. She wanted to have the kind of family she grew up in. Those hopes ended when she finally faced the fact that she was chronically ill.

Jenny ended 1985 the way she started it: hospitalized every month for the same pain she had suffered for eight years. We wanted so badly for the pain to end. Little did we know that her release would come just two months later, in the worst possible way.

6

Ignorance Wasn't Bliss

*The brevity of our life, the dullness of our senses,
the torpor of our indifference, the futility of our occupation,
suffer us to know but little.*
                                              John of Salisbury, 1160

A New Year

"I think you're looking better and getting better, Jenny." She began 1986 with improved test results, and at this regular check-up, Dr. Barber was pleased. By the first of February, though, Jenny called Rosemarie and told her she had been nauseous and vomiting for three days.

"Paulie has the flu," she said, "and I think maybe I've caught it."

Paul took her to see Dr. Barber at Kaiser Hospital emergency room the next day. Her temperature, pulse, and lab tests were normal, so the doctor agreed that it probably was the flu, although he conceded the possibility of a bowel obstruction. He sent her home with instructions to continue her TPN nutrients, Valium and Dilaudid. He called Jenny the next day to see how she was doing, and she told him she was feeling a bit better.

Jenny still wasn't feeling well several days later when Rosemarie suggested a change of scenery and activity might do her some good. They decided to attend a local TV station program where a local psychic was to appear. The waiting line was long, though; they couldn't get in, so they came on to our house, where Lou and I, Paul, and Paulie had waited, expecting to tape the program.

Two days later, on Sunday, Rosemarie and two friends made the trip to San Francisco again to attend a makeover show at the same television station. During the warm-up before the show, one of the station staff announced that a faith healer by the name of Grace 'N Vessel ("Amazing Grace") would be on the show in three weeks. Only two tickets were still available. Rosemarie raised her hand and got them. She and Jenny made plans to attend together, but by the time the show date came, Jenny was seriously ill in the hospital.

The Flu or Not the Flu?

When Rosemarie visited her on February 12, Jenny was in bed and feeling weak. She looked sick. Later that day her condition got worse. Jenny again visited the clinic at Kaiser, complaining of fever and chills. Her temperature had risen to 103 degrees. Paulie still had the flu, and Dr. Barber believed that her symptoms were caused either by the flu or by catheter sepsis (an infection from the catheter). He ordered a blood culture, which turned out negative, and her white blood count was in the normal range. Since these tests did not indicate infection, he concluded again that it was the flu.

Once again, Dr. Barber called Jenny the next day, and once again she reported that she felt a little better. "I will be out of town next week, starting February 16, but I have discussed your case with Dr. Mary Harris, another gastroenterologist here at Kaiser, so she will be standing by in case of any problems," he said.

Dr. Barber's absence may not have been a problem if Jenny had been in the care of a home TPN team whose members had been properly trained to deal with her condition.

It also may have been no problem if Dr. Barber, who Jenny trusted so completely, had left special instructions in her records, so that when emergency care became necessary Dr.

Harris would be called for consultation.

Unfortunately, no one at the emergency room knew her special needs, although they had access to all her records. And without Dr. Barber's notations, no one from the emergency room ever called on Dr. Harris for a consultation. None of the Kaiser emergency room physicians had experience with the Hickman catheter, and they had apparently had no idea how to diagnose possible catheter infections.

So there was Jenny at home, her fever rising and her condition deteriorating. Although she had been hospitalized before for catheter infections, no one had been alerted about her condition. No one on staff was trained to diagnose a catheter infection. It was a dangerous situation.

Jenny spent the next day at home in bed, while the family worried about her. She mumbled while she was on the phone with me. Rosemarie went grocery shopping for her and bought Popsicles and simple things Jenny could fix for herself.

"She does look like she has the flu," Rosemarie said, but we were worried because she was slurring her words and seemed to slip in and out of delirium. Sometimes she sounded as if she were speaking a foreign language. She had a fever that night. We knew something was very wrong.

On Saturday, the 15th, Jenny called to tell me her fever was up to 104 degrees. I told Paul to rub her down with alcohol. When I called her back that evening, her fever was down.

Rosemarie called Jenny that day and noticed that her speech was slurring. It was hard to understand her.

Late that night, her Hickman developed hairline cracks in two places while she was irrigating (cleaning) it. Paul noticed that the line was leaking near the heparin port. He saw what looked like condensation at the bottom of the tube. When Jenny realized that the catheter had been damaged, she clamped the line shut. Paul called the emergency room at Kaiser.

The response was, "Bring her in tomorrow morning, and we'll take a look at it."

On Sunday, Paul took her in as instructed. They checked her temperature, which was slightly elevated, at 99.8 degrees. Her pulse was tachycardic (elevated), and she continued to have flu-like symptoms. They took no blood cultures.

"Mom, Jenny looks terrible," Rosemarie said. "and she can't speak above a whisper."

She told Rosemarie that she had a "blown line" (a break in her Hickman catheter). The emergency room doctor thought she had the flu. They repaired the catheter and sent her home again.

We had no way of knowing it then, but the emergency room physician was unable to draw any blood from the catheter either before or after the repair. This might indicate that a small blood clot had formed in the Hickman catheter. If so, that clot could have been the perfect place for bacteria to grow.

On Monday, Rosemarie called Kaiser. The hospital staff said that there was no one to talk to, since Dr. Barber was on vacation. The family was now seriously concerned that Jenny's problem was not just the flu. When I talked to Jenny on the phone, her speech was slurred, and she said that she was feverish. Paul said that she was confused and very thirsty. Her coordination was altered.

"She took a whole pitcher of water and poured it down the front of her pants while she was standing at the sink," Paul said

We wanted to believe that it was just the flu, but deep in our hearts we knew better. Her primary care physician was gone, and no one offered any suggestions about what to do. We wanted to share our concerns with someone, but whom?

Jenny called the nursing service and told the nurse taking the call that she had continued to use the line after the breach. The nurse told her to call back to the emergency room if there were any signs of the catheter not functioning properly.

When Josephine Caplan, R.N., the home health care nurse, visited Jenny on Tuesday, February 18, she found her weak, exhausted, and with a 102-degree fever. Rosemarie took Jenny home with her that afternoon. She said, "As Jenny sat at my kitchen table, she still looked very sick. I noticed that she was putting an unusual amount of sugar in her coffee. She was also slurring her words."

Jenny insisted she was feeling better, and that she just had the flu. Rosemarie knew that the home health care nurse, a medical professional, had just seen her, so she didn't panic.

On the 19th family members were all on the phone with each other, discussing Jenny's condition. She continued to insist it was just the flu, but we were afraid. All the warning flags were up. Jenny wasn't improving. None of the medical people were doing anything.

Rosemarie called the visiting nurse's office to find out when the next visit would take place. They said it would be the following Tuesday, six days away. I was worried that Jenny wasn't getting a complete checkup, and I told them to notify me when the nurse was going to arrive so that I could be there.

A Downhill Spiral

Paul called Rosemarie the next day and told her that Jenny's blood sugar was only 37 (too low). Rosemarie called the visiting nurse's office and told Ms. Caplan that she was concerned about Jenny's deteriorating condition. She repeated that Jenny had been sick for a week and that she had experienced a blown line. She mentioned that the line had been repaired at Kaiser, that she had been evaluated, and that they had sent her home.

"What? I can't believe they would send her home after she had a blown line!" Ms. Caplan said. This, after all, was an event that was potentially life threatening. "Take her back to the hospital right away for a re-evaluation."

We lost no time following through with this recommendation. Rosemarie picked up Paul and Jennifer at their house. Jenny was pale, delirious, slurring her words and was so weak she could hardly get dressed. Rosemarie headed for Kaiser as soon as they could get Jenny in the car.

As she lay on a gurney (a wheeled stretcher) at the hospital, Rosemarie and others fired questions at her, and Jenny tried to answer. Sometimes she started talking to people who weren't there; then suddenly she would be fine again. When Rosemarie asked her about it, Jenny said, "I must have been dreaming.

Jenny told Dr. Thompson in the emergency room that she had experienced a fever of up to 102 degrees since the previous Thursday. While she was at Kaiser that morning she had a temperature of 97 degrees, her speech was slurred, and she was delirious and had poor physical coordination. Her pulse raced at 120 beats per minute and her white blood count was up to 15,600, fifty percent above normal. In addition, her serum glucose levels were markedly elevated.

Dr. Thompson questioned Rosemarie and Jenny about her

symptoms. Thompson, who was unfamiliar with Jenny's case, thought the delirium could be related to the painkiller Dilaudid. "No," Rosemarie told him. "Jenny has been on these pain medications for a long time, and I have never ever seen her act like this. There is something wrong."

He gave Rosemarie a look that made it clear that he didn't believe her. Meanwhile, the delirious Jenny kept repeating, "It's just the flu. I don't want to go into the hospital again."

Had Dr. Thompson been properly trained, he would have known that Jenny's tachycardia, delirium, high temperature and high serum glucose levels were warning signs of catheter infection. He didn't.

Because he was uncertain how to diagnose her condition, he called for a second opinion from Dr. Nicholas Scott, a specialist in internal medicine. He put Jenny on an intravenous drip to replenish her body fluids. Since it was time for Paulie to get out of school, Rosemarie and Paul left to pick him up, and Rosemarie drove them home. She then drove the 16 miles to her own house to await news from the hospital.

Dr. Scott examined Jenny, took a blood culture and called Rosemarie early that afternoon. "It appears to be a combination of her blood sugars, her fever and the flu," he said.

"Just keep her fever down and continue with her normal medications. I'll prescribe some Tylenol suppositories for the fever." In his Emergency Room Consultation Record, Dr. Scott's diagnosis was "viral syndrome with *no evidence of localized infection or catheter sepsis.*"

Rosemarie was dismayed. "I offered her hospitalization, but she doesn't want to stay," Dr. Scott told her. "Besides, there is little we can do in the hospital that she can't do at home. I saw no signs of catheter-related problems."

Rosemarie wasn't at all certain that Jenny knew what the doctor was saying. She said to Dr. Scott, "She has no business going home. She can't even talk."

Dr. Scott left it up to her. He said that if Jenny didn't want to stay, they couldn't keep her. Rosemarie wanted Jenny to stay because she was delirious. She felt that they didn't understand her condition and that the doctor really thought it best for her to stay in the hospital. Jenny wanted to leave.

The real problem was this: Jenny didn't have the flu. Dr. Thompson and Dr. Scott were both wrong. Dead wrong. Jenny was already in the midst of catheter sepsis: a serious infection originating from the site where the catheter enters her body. Catheter sepsis is one of the primary complications of inpatient or home TPN. Because of the speed at which the infection can spread, catheter infections must be treated in an aggressive manner. If not recognized and treated quickly, the infection can quickly lead to death.

The earliest symptom of catheter sepsis is a fever. Jenny's temperature was 102 degrees on the 20th; it had been that high periodically for over a week. As the sepsis progresses to the second stage, symptoms include tachycardia (Jenny's heart rate was high at 120 and more), altered mental status (Jenny was delirious), an elevated white blood count (Jenny's was up over 50 percent), hyperglycemia, rapid breathing, and blood pressure disorders. If discovered and aggressively treated in this stage, the patient has a fair chance of recovery. In its third stage, when the patient has barely a fighting chance of survival, the infection leads to altered renal (kidney) function, disordered coagulation, and impaired lung function. The final stage is cardiovascular collapse (heart stoppage) and eventually death. It is clear that by the 20th Jenny was already well into the second stage of catheter sepsis.

By 1986, experts in TPN had known for nearly fifteen years that catheter patients like Jenny needed special monitoring. They also knew that any catheter patient with a fever should be automatically assumed to have catheter sepsis unless the fever could be clearly explained by some other process. With all Jenny's medical records available and her long history of catheter problems, the Kaiser staff should have been able to diagnose and treat her infection. As we know now, they didn't have a clue. But we didn't know that at the time.

When Rosemarie told me that the doctors at Kaiser thought her delusions were from a flu-induced fever, we were both greatly relieved. "Thank you, Dear Lord, for letting it be just a case of the flu," I remember thinking. When Rosemarie went to pick her up, Jenny was sitting in a wheelchair. She had regained a little bit of color in her face, and she was more coherent.

Jenny said to Rosemarie, "Oh, God. You'll never believe what happened. I asked for something to drink and they gave me some orange juice. I guess I must have spilled some. Then they told me I could get dressed and go home. I was stepping off the gurney onto a step stool. I must have slipped on the juice. I fell and landed on my hip."

Rosemarie was shocked. She said to herself, "*What on earth are these people doing, leaving a weak, delirious girl alone like that?*" She asked Jenny, "Did you tell anyone?"

"Yes," Jenny said. "The nurse looked at it. She said it was just a bruise and that I was okay."

Rosemarie asked, "Did they take any x-rays?"

"No," Jenny replied.

Although her hip was hurting, she didn't want to spend a single unnecessary minute in the hospital, and she asked Rosemarie to take her home. When they reached Jenny's home, Paul had to carry her into the house.

That afternoon, Rosemarie spoke with Jenny on the telephone and noticed that she was slurring her speech again. That evening, Vince came to visit Rosemarie and she had him call Jenny's home to talk with her. Vince dialed the number, and Jenny answered, but she couldn't identify her brother's voice. She mumbled and slurred her words, and what she said didn't make sense. Vince turned to his sister and said, "Rosemarie, something is wrong!" He was very alarmed.

All that night, Jenny's hip hurt badly, and her speech was slurred again. She did not move from the couch all night, even to use the bathroom. She wet the couch that night.

Jenny came to stay at Rosemarie's house the next day. She still had the fever and was feeling worse overall. Now, because of her hip pain, she couldn't walk. Rosemarie saw that she was deteriorating.

"Maybe if I give you a warm bath you'll feel better," she said.

"No, I'm afraid it will hurt my legs too much," Jenny said. She chose instead to have Rosemarie bathe her feet and put her hair up in braids. Because of the pain in her hip, Rosemarie had to help Jenny to the bathroom, as she couldn't make it alone.

Jenny was desperately thirsty all day and the whole night. She drank Coke after Coke and glass after glass of water.

Rosemarie took her temperature every hour and gave her Tylenol. She was delirious off and on all day. She would be talking to Rosemarie or Paul one minute, and then she would suddenly doze off and start mumbling and talking to people who weren't there. Minutes later she would be lucid again, making complete sense.

Rosemarie put Jenny in her daughter's room, and when it came time for Jenny to hook up the TPN medication pump to her Hickman catheter, she was too weak to do it. Rosemarie didn't know how to operate the TPN pump. She did know that turning on the wrong switch could blow the line again. Jenny was too weak to explain the complicated procedure, so she went without her nutrition and medications that night. Rosemarie didn't want Jenny to be alone, so she slept in the other bed in her daughter's room. Neither of them slept much that night.

Rosemarie knew that something was terribly wrong. So did Jenny. About sunrise, Jenny turned to Rosemarie and said, "I love you."

Rosemarie took her hand and replied, "I love you too, Jenny."

7

Amazing Grace

Is there no pity in the clouds
that sees the bottom of my grief?
Shakespeare, *Romeo and Juliet*

Infection, Pneumonia, and a Broken Hip

"Well, I don't know Jenny," Jean, a Kaiser nurse said on the telephone, "but from what I understand she likes to stay pretty well snowed." It was Saturday morning, February 22, and Rosemarie was worried sick about Jenny's deteriorating condition. She slammed down the receiver. This statement represented the Kaiser attitude. To them, Jenny was just an addict who used her condition to get drugs.

Jean had already told Rosemarie that she checked Jenny's records and there was no mention of her falling in the emergency room, that her blood culture was fine, and that Dr. Thompson said the delirium was probably caused by her painkiller, Dilauded.

Jenny felt terrible. Her feet were swelling, and she was unable to use the bathroom without assistance. Rosemarie brought her a bedpan to use, but left the door to her room open, because there was no one around. Jenny said to Rosemarie, "Close that door. There's people there."

Rosemarie said, "Jenny, there's no one there."

"Oh, okay," she replied. She was hallucinating again, and Rosemarie was afraid for her.

Rosemarie thought Jenny may have broken her hip in her fall at the hospital, and Jenny agreed. Rosemarie was worried about pneumonia, too, plus the fact that Jenny hadn't been able to hook up her TPN machine and take her medications the night before.

She helped Jenny out of bed and into her kitchen. When she made some tomato soup, one of Jenny's favorite foods, Jenny couldn't eat it. She would be talking to Rosemarie and then suddenly start talking to people who weren't there. The delirium continued.

Just after noon, Rosemarie got a phone call from Dr. David Proctor, the physician on call at Kaiser that day. He told her to immediately bring Jenny back in for reevaluation.

"Something has come up on her blood test," he said.

Her blood test? At ten o'clock that same morning, the nurse from the Kaiser emergency room had told us that there was nothing wrong with her blood test and that her problems were probably from the Dilaudid. We were actually relieved. Finally, there was a reason for her delirium: Jenny's got an infection. That's what is causing it.

Jenny couldn't walk, and felt she couldn't sit up in a wheelchair. Rosemarie told the emergency room they were on the way in, and asked them to have a gurney waiting. Bob, Rosemarie's husband, picked up Jenny and carried her to the car. She drifted in and out of delirium during the short drive to Kaiser. She didn't like the news about the possible infection—but within seconds, she had lost touch with reality again and didn't know she was on the way to the hospital.

We were actually glad that they were admitting her again, because we thought they'd figure out the problem, give her medications and discharge her.

They drove to the emergency room, went in and told them that Jennifer was there. The nurse brought a wheelchair. Jenny said, "I don't think I can get into the wheelchair."

The nurse said to her, "It's just as easy for you to get into a wheelchair as onto a gurney."

Rosemarie didn't want to argue with the nurse. She just wanted Jenny admitted to the hospital. They took her directly to an examination room. Paul met Rosemarie and Jenny there. The hospital personnel finally brought a gurney and laid Jenny down on it. The three of them sat in that room for two and a half hours, waiting for someone to come and see Jenny.

They waited and waited. And they kept thinking: *Don't make a scene. The doctor is busy somewhere with other patients.* Jenny had to relieve herself. She couldn't move on her own, had no one to help her, had nowhere to go, and went on the gurney. With the interminable wait, —she finally had to go. Rosemarie was so angry. No one should be treated this way, she felt. In desperation, Rosemarie went out and found a nurse. She told the woman how long Jenny had been waiting and suffering.

Finally Dr. Proctor came in. He was very gentle with her. He asked her if she knew her name, what day it was, and who the president of the United States was. Jenny got all three wrong. She was delirious. Jenny's pulse was racing at 148 beats per minute, and her breathing was rapid. Dr. Proctor had her admitted immediately and ordered an x-ray of her hip. Rosemarie was relieved, and went home to get some sleep.

That evening when she returned, Rosemarie learned that Jenny had a fractured hip and a raging infection caused by two deadly types of bacteria: *staphylococcus aureus lactamase* and *streptococcus viridens.* In addition, a chest x-ray showed severe problems in both lungs: she was developing pneumonia.

Jenny was started on aggressive antibiotic therapy to treat her catheter infection. But unknown to us, the Kaiser physicians were treating her with antibiotics that the doctors at Memorial Hospital had already found to be ineffective on her and had carefully noted in her medical records. It was another deadly oversight by Kaiser.

Despite her symptoms, the alarming clinical information, positive blood cultures and previous history of catheter infections, the doctors at Kaiser chose not to remove the Hickman catheter for two more days. This decision flew in the face of all logic (except the logic of money). The Kaiser physicians knew that if they removed the catheter, they would likely have to replace it later with another one (at a cost of about $10,000). Even though it was infected, they evidently tried to delay removing the catheter and thereby save Kaiser the cost of putting in a new one.

A week later, when Dr. Barber returned and found that Jenny had experienced two holes in her line, he said he would have hospitalized her immediately. He also said that he would have immediately removed the catheter when it was obvious that it was infected. Those two decisions, not to admit her when the catheter was broken and the delay in removing the infected catheter, further compromised Jenny's chance of survival.

Dr. Barber later made a shocking revelation to Jenny's husband, Paul. The Kaiser physician told him that he had been worried that Jenny wouldn't get proper care while he was gone. "No one at Kaiser wants to treat her because she is so sick," he said. He said he had indeed ordered Jenny's medicines in advance, because "No one wanted to treat her unless they had to."

When Rosemarie visited Jenny on Sunday, she was resting better, but her situation was deteriorating. An x-ray showed that she had a fractured hip. The hospital staff tried to convince Rosemarie that Jenny had fallen in the tub at home, which made Rosemarie angry. It seemed as though everyone at Kaiser was trying to duck the blame for what they permitted to happen to Jenny or made her endure.

Rosemarie, who had spent the most time helping Jenny get care, was particularly upset. When Jenny was admitted to the ICU (intensive care unit), she went to see Dr. Barber. "I don't like one bit the way she's being treated," she said. "I want to talk about this."

"I don't want to talk about it now," he replied.

"There are some things I want to complain about," Rosemarie continued.

"When this thing is over and she's out of intensive care, we're going to talk." Dr. Barber agreed.

Rosemarie was in constant touch with all the family members. Lou and I, who were still living in San Francisco, arranged to drive to San Rafael the next day.

A 50/50 Chance

I saw Jenny in her room at Kaiser on Monday. Shortly after I arrived, the doctors told me that her condition was worsening and that the prognosis wasn't good. They said that she had only a 50/50 chance to live. Dr. Barber had just returned from vacation. He told us that the infection had invaded Jenny's lungs and pneumonia was setting in. She was quickly transferred to the intensive care unit. There, the Hickman line, which was the source of her infection, was finally removed. I immediately notified all the family so that they could come to the hospital as soon as possible.

Vince was at work when I called him. He left for the hospital immediately. By Monday night, the whole family had assembled in the hospital. The pneumonia was making breathing difficult for Jenny. They had placed an oxygen mask on her by then, but she was still gasping for breath. She was suffering longer and longer periods of delirium and was barely able to communicate. We spent that night giving her ice chips to soothe her dry lips and thirst.

The Kaiser staff decided that she should immediately be put on a respirator to help her breathe. Jenny sensed that this would make it even harder for her to communicate with us, and she wanted her family to be with her.

We entered her room, and Lou stood at the head of her bed. When he saw how she suffered, he broke down in tears and had to leave her room. Although Jenny was suffering intense pain, she immediately thought of comforting her father. She told Rosemarie, "Go check on Dad. I'm worried about him."

Cathy remembers arriving at the waiting room after Jenny was put on the respirator. "I sat next to my Dad and started to cry, because they had already put her on the life support equipment before I had a chance to talk to her. I remember my Dad trying to comfort me as he did when I was a little girl. He took his hand and gently rubbed my whole face, as if to say, 'Don't worry, everything's going to be OK.' "

Jenny had a raging infection, and she was burning up with heat. Her diabetes was also out of control. One doctor evidently thought that her changing blood sugar level was from an undocumented infusion of glucose in the emergency room. It wasn't. The glucose increase was a sign of the infection that they had overlooked. It was awful seeing her like that, because we all knew that her condition was very serious. We hoped that with her own enormous inner strength and God's help, Jenny would pull through, but at some level, we knew that she might not. As Jenny had always done, we chose to see the glass as half full, rather than half empty.

This crisis started the countdown that would last for a week. By Monday night, the pneumonia was making breathing difficult for her. They were giving her oxygen through a mask, but she was still gasping for breath. She was coherent, but extremely weak. The doctor had told us that they might put her on a respirator in order to take the load off her lungs. We were all terrified. I stayed at Rosemarie's house that night so that I could be close to the hospital. Paul stayed with Jenny in her room.

At some point that week Dr. Barber felt that she had made a slight improvement, and he told us that her survival chances had risen to 70/30. That really raised our spirits (for an hour or two).

At 4:00 A.M. Thursday Paul called and told us that they were putting Jenny on a respirator. She was going through an agonizing struggle. We dressed immediately and reached the hospital within a half hour.

Jenny was looking much worse. She was sitting up in bed struggling for breath. Her face was flushed. All she could say to us was, "I'm so tired."

For the rest of the week, she was sedated, but she tried to talk with us. Cathy, Rosemarie and I stayed with her all the time. We tried to cheer her up and make her as comfortable as possible. She couldn't move her head or hands much, but she managed to mouth words. She told each of us, "I love you." It took a great effort on her part to say anything.

Vince recalls that when he saw her that week she was heavily sedated. She was aware of her surroundings, though it seemed like she was asleep. He would squeeze her hand, and when she could, she would give a gentle squeeze back.

Each day she was on the respirator, more fluid collected in her body. By this time she had swollen to grotesque proportions.

That last week of Jenny's life the entire family was in constant prayer for Jenny. We only had our faith and each other to get us through. I went to church or visited the hospital chapel every day, and I remember Cathy coming to church with me, kneeling in front of the Blessed Mother, lighting a candle and praying for Jenny.

When Jenny's sisters and brother look back and talk about those horrible last days, each of them remembers different things. Cathy remembers the sound of the respirator. Every time she heard it, she thought, "Oh no. That's Jenny's last breath." She also remembers that when you walked into Jenny's room, the first thing you saw were the x-rays, which were illuminated by light boxes attached to the wall. That reminded you of what was going on inside that poor girl's body. Rosemarie remembers the anti-septic smell of the emergency room and the smell of surgical tape made wet by saliva. They use the tape to stabilize the respirator tube in the patient's mouth.

On Wednesday, Jenny's condition had not improved. The doctor inserted a catheter into one of her arteries that day, and the next day he placed a Swann Ganz catheter in her right femoral vein.

Her infection raged out of control. Her body temperature was so high that they put her on an ice blanket. She wore only a short hospital gown, and she complained about feeling cold. We watched her shiver. Inside she was burning up; outside she was shivering. It was torture for Jenny, but also very hard on us. Jenny always slept with socks on, so we asked the intensive care nurse, whose name was Rhonda, if they would allow that. She said that would be all right, and we put her socks on. They also let us cover her with a light sheet, which seemed to make her a little more comfortable.

Amazing Grace

Jenny had a slow, horrible death. The only one at Kaiser who was truly good to Jenny was Rhonda. She was kind, gentle, thoughtful, and went out of her way to be nice to Jenny. She spent a lot of time with her, and was always sensitive to her needs. She would say in a gentle voice, "Jenny? Is there anything I can do for you?"

That morning, Amazing Grace, the faith healer, was on the "People Are Talking Show," and Lou decided to watch her. He wasn't the type of person to put much credence in faith healers, but he did believe that you could cure yourself if you had the right frame of mind. When he came to the hospital later in the day, I asked him if he had seen the program. He said yes, and that he was impressed. He also said that she was going to appear at the Palace of Fine Arts in San Francisco on Saturday night, March 1.

By Friday night, we were all very tired. We had been at the hospital all day visiting Jenny and had returned to Rosemarie's house to rest. The phone rang. It was Rhonda, the ICU nurse. She told Rosemarie, "Come back to the hospital. I can't put my finger on what's happening, but Jenny is going within herself. I think she really needs to see you."

Jenny was relieved to see us, and felt much better because we were there. She was very restless for a time; then her eyes started to look glassy. She became quiet, and didn't respond much. Rhonda noticed and pointed it out to us.

Her sisters had noticed the final decline in her spirit earlier that day. Cathy and Rosemarie had gone into her room and said to her, "You're looking better, Jenny. We're going to put you on a gurney, sneak you out of here, and take you home." Jenny raised her leg a little and moved it from side to side. That meant no.

As we look back on it now, Jenny was telling us that she was going to be leaving us. That night, Lou decided that he was going to see Amazing Grace in person.

The night of the show, the family was all with Jenny in the hospital. After Lou visited with her for a while, he left with Paulie to see Amazing Grace. Like the rest of us, Lou was desperate to get Jenny some help. He knew that his daughter was critically ill. He didn't know what to do, but he knew he had to do something. The faith healer seemed like the last hope.

He had seen faith healers before. Lou was no fool. He wasn't the kind to be taken in by quacks or showmen. But he was a man without a lot of choices, and he undoubtedly thought, *What can it hurt?* Jenny was chronically ill. All the medical people in her life couldn't stop her pain. I'm sure he thought that maybe, if you have enough faith, there might be someone who can reach God better than you can. If intense faith can help, why not use it?

Grace was a young woman in her early thirties from Brookfield, Connecticut. She did most of her work in New

England. This was to be her first and last healing service in San Francisco. Other than what we saw on the television show, we didn't know anything about her.

With the exception of the Rev. Billy Graham, Lou never had much respect for television preachers or faith healers, but Grace got his attention. He liked how she presented herself. Maybe it was her, or maybe it was his desperation. We don't know. In any case, he decided to go see her healing service at the Palace of Fine Arts at 7:30 that night. Lou was clearly hoping for some kind of miracle.

He left the hospital about 5:30 PM with our grandson Paulie. He didn't have advance tickets for the show, and they stood in line for two hours to get in. About 11:30 that night, Lou called us and described what had happened.

After Grace had explained how she felt God's healing power worked, she asked the audience if there was anyone who wanted her to pray for a loved one. She also said that she would be happy to bless anything they would like blessed. She would come down each aisle, she said, and whoever wanted to tell of a prayer need or receive a blessing should come forward.

When she came down Lou's aisle he held out the handkerchief. "Please bless this," he said. "I have a daughter who is critically ill." Grace quickly blessed the handkerchief and moved on to the next person. Then, after she had passed along and spoken with several other people, she turned around and returned to Lou.

Grace seemed to know something that we didn't. She looked Lou straight in the eye and blessed him, and then she did the same for Paulie. Amazing Grace said to Lou, "Your daughter will never have to suffer again, and her father will never leave her."

8

Daddy Will Never Leave You

The bustle in a house
The morning after death
Is solemnest of industries
Enacted upon earth.
The sweeping up the heart,
And putting love away
We shall not want to use again
Until eternity.
                                        Emily Dickinson

Sunday, March 2, 1986

The anxiety level in the intensive care unit waiting room was excruciating as our family prayed for the life of my daughter, Jennifer Gigliello.

That morning we all gathered at the hospital, praying for the best and fearing the worst. Jenny was heavily sedated. Most of the time she looked as if she were asleep. We would talk to her, and she would communicate by squeezing our hand. One squeeze for yes, two for no. That's all she could do. I choked back my own tears as I tried to swallow the lump in my throat. "Be strong for the children," I told myself.

When Lou came in, he carried the handkerchief that had been blessed by Amazing Grace. Vince recalls that Lou went straight over to Jenny. Her face perspired, and her hair was very damp. Lou wiped her face with the handkerchief. He said to Jenny, "This is from Amazing Grace. She said, 'Christ said that you will never have to suffer.' Don't worry. Your Daddy will never leave you." That was his way of comforting her.

The last time I saw Lou like that was when his mother was in the hospital. It was as if he had tuned everybody else out, and he was the healer. It showed us all how much love he had for his daughter. He tried to put the handkerchief in Jenny's hand, but she was too weak to hold it. We had the nurse pin it to her pillow near her head, along with a note not to remove it.

By that afternoon we needed a break and some food. At Rosemarie's house, while we were eating, Lou went to the telephone and called Amazing Grace's prayer counseling line. He stayed on for almost an hour. Turning to a faith healer for spiritual consolation was out of character for Lou, but it showed the depth of his despair. He was a smart, self-reliant man who researched the answers to his own questions and didn't turn to others unless he had exhausted his own resources.

Lou seemed greatly comforted by the time he spent on the prayer line. It helped make it easier for him to cope with Jenny's critical condition. When he was through, we all went back to the hospital.

Everyone was sitting in the intensive care waiting room about 6:30 that night when they called a "Code Blue," meaning that someone had gone into cardiac arrest. We had just come out of her room. Rosemarie knew that it was Jenny, yet she didn't say anything to me because she hoped she was wrong. She didn't have to say anything. I took one look at Rosemarie's face and knew something bad was happening. Rosemarie turned as white as a sheet. It was as if the spirit of life had left her.

I saw all these people rushing into Jenny's room. I was praying, "Don't let it be Jenny." But immediately I realized that it was my daughter they were trying to revive.

The staff started cardiac resuscitation. Vince opened the door and saw all the people in her room. Lou got up and went outside on the patio near the intensive care unit and walked around. He could see into the ICU from an outside window, and he reported to us that they were pumping on her chest, performing CPR (cardiopulmonary resuscitation).

A short time later, Dr. Mary Harris came and told us that Jenny had experienced a cardiac arrest. "We were able to bring her back," she said enthusiastically. "She has some color in her face again. Her lungs collapsed. We don't know what the outcome will be, but she's a fighter."

Cathy remembers looking through the glass doors of the waiting room out onto a patio. Rosemarie and Vince were hugging each other and crying. Inside the waiting room, Lou and I were comforting each other.

Dr. Harris said we could go in and see her. We were all so relieved that they had been able to revive her. However, our joy and relief was short-lived. As soon as we looked at Jenny, we knew that her spirit had already left her. She still had a pulse and the respirator was making it possible for her to breathe, but the Jenny we knew was gone.

Monday, March 3, 1986

A Catholic priest had already been called by the hospital and had given Jenny the last rites of the Church the day before, but we hadn't been there to take part. On Monday we asked him to come again so that the family could participate. He arrived about 10:00 a.m., and the ceremony was held at her bedside.

On Monday morning, Kaiser's Dr. Henry C. Barber called us all together and told us the bad news. Jenny was in the worst condition possible; her body was alive but she was brain dead.

Then came the hard question: what to do if she went into cardiac arrest again. Did we want them to try to revive her?

We were tortured with that decision. Most of us had accepted the fact that the Jenny we knew was no longer with us. Paul wanted her revived if she arrested again. He was terrified of losing his wife, and he was angry that Dr. Thompson had failed to admit her on the 20th, when there might still have been a chance of saving her life. Paul wanted to go down to the emergency room and physically attack Dr. Thompson for his negligence. Lou restrained him and calmed him down. He said, "Don't go down there. It won't solve anything. Just leave it alone. When this is all over, we'll take care of it."

In a few minutes the neurologist arrived to examine Jenny. A short time later, we heard those dreadful words again: Code Blue.

This time, Dr. Harris and the ICU staff calmly walked in and went through the motions. After a few minutes, they turned off all the screaming monitors and disconnected the life support equipment. They couldn't bring her back again. Jenny was dead, the victim of eight years of misdiagnosis, needless operations, incompetence, and neglect.

Hospitals deal with the death of patients and the effect of death on the surviving families every day. Most hospitals try to minimize the trauma to the family when a death occurs. Before the family is admitted to see the deceased patient, the hospital takes at least some basic steps so the sight that greets the grieving family isn't any more traumatic than absolutely necessary. Tubes and bloodstained dressings are removed, and open wounds are covered. The patient's body is arranged in a peaceful sleeping position. A physician explains to the family how the end came and offers condolences.

No one at Kaiser bothered to perform any of those things for Jenny or our family.

When Lou and I were told we could have a few private moments with Jenny, we went into her room and were shocked at how we found her. It looked as though she had been shoved into the side of the bed. Her head was hanging half over the side. A trickle of blood was running down from the edge of her mouth. She looked like a rag doll that had been tossed aside. Doctors and nurses wandered through the ICU ward, ignoring us and talking to each other as if we were not there and nothing unusual had happened. It was obvious that they didn't care about us or Jenny.

As Lou and I came out of the room, Rosemarie, Vince and Cathy were about to go in. Lou advised against it. He didn't want them to see her like that.

We left the room. I wanted to scream with rage. I started to break down. Lou knew what was going on. He patted me on the arm to say, "Hold on a little bit longer, Dorothy. We need to be strong for the children's sake."

Paulie wanted to go in and see his mom. He was yelling and crying because we didn't want him to see her in that condition, and we had to physically restrain him.

No one lifted a finger to spare our feelings. No one even said that they were sorry that our daughter had died. No one attempted to explain anything or console us. Not even Dr. Barber. He went to his desk and started writing out his reports, as though we didn't exist. I think the entire staff at Kaiser was glad to be rid of her.

At 1:30 PM on Monday, March 3, 1986, Jenny Gigliello died of catheter sepsis, bacterial infection and its results: pneumonia, a collapsed lung, two cardiac arrests and sixteen hours of brain death. She was four days short of her thirtieth birthday.

We were all grieving when we left Kaiser Foundation Hospital. As many trips as she had made to the hospital in the past, Jenny had always come home in two or ten or thirty days. This time she wouldn't come home. How could this have happened? How could our family go on without Jenny?

The whole family was in shock, thank God. Shock serves a useful purpose. It insulates you from the awful reality of death long enough to let you do what you need to do.

The week she was in the hospital, we all saw death coming, but I never accepted the fact that she would actually die. I remember sitting in the waiting room, giving her a chance to rest, thinking that if she rested, she'd get better and recover. She'd pull through it, because she'd gone through so many major surgeries and had been in and out of the hospital so many times before. This was just one more time, we thought (or so we tried to convince ourselves). It may have been denial, but denial is as good a way as any to cope with the unthinkable in the short term.

Denial or not, I knew that Jenny was giving up, letting go. After all she had been through, she was tired. It was a very hard death.

Vince drove the car back to my house, because he didn't think Lou was up to it. Cathy sat in front with him, and Lou and I were in the back. Suddenly, the enormity of Jenny's death hit Vince. He began to sob and his body started to shake. Lou reached forward and put his hand on Vince's shoulder. This seemed to calm him. Lou asked him if he was able to drive, and Vince nodded that he could. He recovered his composure and was able to finish driving the family home.

When we arrived home, we all collapsed. Rosemarie told Lou that Jenny's death had been a release from pain, a small miracle in its own right. Lou responded that death wasn't the miracle he'd been praying for.

With Jenny's death a cold reality, we all pulled together as a family and did what we needed to do.

Tuesday, March 4, 1996

Tuesday was Rosemarie's husband Bob's 47th birthday, but we couldn't celebrate it. We had more pressing things to do, arranging Jenny's funeral. Rosemarie and Cathy went with me to Valenti Marini Mortuary in San Francisco the next day and made the final arrangements for Jenny. It took the better part of the day to discuss everything and make all the choices. We were worried about having the casket open because Jenny had been so bloated when she died. The mortuary assistant assured us that Jenny would look like her normal self when the time came for the viewing. Next we took the mortuary elevator downstairs and picked out the casket and the clothes she would be buried in. That was difficult for me to do. Then we returned home and told Lou about what we had chosen.

That afternoon Jenny's godmother came to visit and brought flowers. In a short time visitors started arriving at the house to pay their respects and bring food and flowers.

Wednesday, March 5, 1986

Lou and I went to Holy Cross Cemetery to pick out a burial plot for Jenny. When we talked to the cemetery director, Lou said that he wanted a family plot where the family members could be together. I didn't think this was the best solution, because our children all had their own families. In addition, the plot we were shown was too far in the back of the cemetery to visit easily, and I didn't want to have to walk over other graves to reach the site.

Instead, we chose a sunny spot with benches nearby where we could sit when we came to visit her. Once that decision had been made, Lou said to me, "Since we're here, we should look into getting our own plots close to Jenny. Otherwise, there may not be any when we want them." I agreed. We went back to the mortuary office to sign the deeds to the lots. Lou picked up the pen to sign them, but then he handed it to me and said, "I think you should sign." I said, "OK," but I thought it was an odd request. I signed the papers, and we left and went home.

Rosemarie recalls, "I decided for some reason that I was going to go with my daughter, Cindy, and buy a puppy for my nephew, Paulie. I had two things in mind. First, he had just lost his mother. Second, his eighth birthday was on the 10th. We drove to a pet store in Santa Rosa and picked out a poodle. I knew nothing could replace the loss of his mother, but a puppy would be something special for him to love."

In the Catholic faith, the wake service is conducted in two parts. The first night of viewing is usually reserved for the family. On the second night, the priest recites the rosary, a series of prayers to help the soul make the transition from life to afterlife. Friends of the family usually attend the rosary.

That evening was the first night of the wake. We were very relieved that Jenny looked so pretty (just like we knew her before all the medical and surgical madness). The funeral home was full with her friends, and it was a very emotional time.

During the family viewing, we each passed by the casket and paid our respects to Jenny. Little Paulie put a rose in her casket and kissed her on the forehead. Vince recalls, "The reality of her death didn't really hit me until later. There she was in the coffin (I could see that) but it wasn't the person I knew. The emotions came later."

Several weeks later, Paulie had a startling experience at his home in Novato. One evening he walked into the darkened bathroom, and there, right in front of him, he saw a pale apparition. It was Jenny. She was dressed in white, looking vibrant and healthy, and she was smiling at him. Instinctively he turned on the light to see her better, but as soon as he did, she was gone. Alarmed, he ran to the living room and told his father. Paulie had seen apparitions before. One could even say he attracted them. Once when he was about four years old, he was staying with Lou and me. He came running to Lou and said, "Grandpa, there's a woman out there."

Lou said, "Where? I don't see anyone."

Paulie replied, "She came down the stairs."

Lou rose and took a look around. "Nobody's here, Paulie," he said, but Paulie wasn't convinced. He ran upstairs and got Jenny, who was also staying with us at the time. She asked him to describe what he saw.

"It was a little old lady with gray hair, a blue sweater and an apron. She was kind of stooped over." Paulie had never met Lou's mother while she was alive, but he had just described her perfectly.

From the moment of Jenny's death and throughout the coming days, Lou tried hard to be strong. He kept reassuring us and telling us everything would be okay. I don't think he shed any tears that week.

About 8:00 p.m., Cathy was standing just outside the viewing room, talking to the callers, when she noticed that her father seemed to be having a dizzy spell. He lost his balance, then regained it. "Dad, you better sit down," Cathy told him. She knew how emotionally distraught he was.

He sat down and reassured his daughter that he was OK, but Cathy came to me and quietly said, "Mom, keep an eye on Dad tonight. He was feeling dizzy."

Then Cathy said quietly, "Don't turn around..." but it was too late. I had already looked over at Lou, and his eyes met mine. He realized that Cathy had told me about the dizzy spell, and he looked concerned because he didn't want to worry me.

My mother was in her nineties. When she saw Jenny in the casket she went to pieces. "Take her home before she has a heart attack right here," Lou told a relative.

"There's no way I am going to leave," she said. "I'm sitting right here till it's over." Lou was more concerned for his mother-in-law than for himself.

That night, Lou, Paulie and I all slept in one room; we didn't want Paulie to be alone. When I awoke about two o'clock in the morning, Lou was gone from bed. He wanted to be alone with his thoughts, and went to the spare bedroom to sleep.

Thursday, March 6, 1986

The next morning when I went to his room, Lou was sobbing. It was the first time all week that he let himself express his emotions. Later that day, in spite of his sorrow, he went outside and started washing the front of the house with a hose. He invited Paulie to join him, and finished washing the house. Then he came in, went upstairs, and took a shower.

The family met at my house before going on to the rosary. People were still coming by the house to pay their respects. Rosemarie had just arrived, and had brought with her Jenny's obituary in the Marin *Independent Journal*. Lou didn't want to see it. Rosemarie gave him a kiss. Lou was quiet, very within himself.

The rosary started at 7:00 p.m., and we wanted to be there early to be alone with Jenny before the rest of the mourners arrived. While the family waited in the car, Lou was a little late coming down from the house. Paulie later told me what happened then. Usually, when Lou left the house, he would say to Paulie, "See you later, alligator." That night, he said it to Paulie and three of our other grandchildren before he went downstairs. The oldest two were staying behind with the two youngest. When Lou reached the bottom of the stairs, he turned around and came all the way back up. He looked at the children and said, "I love you," and kissed each of them on the forehead. It was as though he had a premonition of something to come.

Lou and I, the children, and three younger grandchildren all rode together to the mortuary. We had planned to bring some of the children to see Jenny at different times that night.

We were the first to enter the viewing room that evening. The open casket had a kneeler placed in front of it, and the room was illuminated by candles and filled with flowers.

We all gathered around the casket. After we said our goodbyes, we took our seats in the front pew. Lou waited. It was clear to me that he was having a hard time keeping his composure. He was the only one at the head of Jenny's casket. The rest of us had already sat down. Lou leaned over Jenny and sobbed. He tenderly kissed her three times on the forehead, then reached for the kneeler. He knelt on it and bowed his head, as if in prayer.

Cathy recalls, "Everything seemed to be happening in slow motion. It seemed as though all the room lights dimmed and

Jennifer was illuminated in the casket. You could feel the warmth from the candles. The colors of the flowers became vibrant. There was an overall feeling of peacefulness. We felt the love between Dad and Jenny. We didn't know until days later that all of us had this spiritual experience at the same time."

Lou still knelt on the kneeler. Then he shook his head a bit, and bowed his head again. We were worried, so we hurried to him. At that moment, he started to fall off the kneeler. We thought he was fainting, and we rushed to his side. He slumped into our arms.

Rosemarie recalls, "The children, Trina, Cindy, and Louie were sitting off to the side. When my father fell over, I knew it wasn't a fainting spell. I jumped up and said to my husband, 'Get the children out of here.'"

We immediately laid Lou on the floor. The special glow from the casket dimmed, and everything seemed gray and dark. Rosemarie, who knew CPR, immediately loosened his tie, cleared his airway, and started to try to resuscitate him.

The scene was pure hysteria. I was yelling that we needed help, and people from other rooms in the mortuary came running to help us.

The mortuary staff called the paramedics, while Rosemarie continued CPR. Lou's eyes were open, and his gaze was fixed. When the paramedics arrived, we left the room. They used shock paddles to try to restart his heart, but it was no use. When they put Lou in the ambulance, Vince got in with him. Our daughters and their husbands followed them to the hospital.

The ambulance driver asked Vince if he had a preference of hospitals. Vince said, "St. Anne's."

"It doesn't look good," the driver told him.

"I remember looking back through the glass window into the back of the ambulance," Vince recalls. "They pumped his chest all the way to the hospital, but I think they were just following procedures. Dad was already gone by then, and I think we all knew that. When we arrived at the hospital, the driver told me to go to the waiting room, where a nurse would meet me. The nurse did everything she could to console me and make me comfortable. She could hardly believe it when I told her my sister had died just three days before.

"Then the emergency room doctor came in and said, 'I'm awfully sorry. Your father didn't make it.' I knew in my heart Dad was gone, but to hear those words brought a reality that I was not ready to accept."

Unlike the heartless treatment we had experienced at Kaiser, the staff at St. Anne's Hospital was very considerate. The nurse advised the children not to go see Lou right away. "He's still hooked up to the equipment," she said. "You might want to wait a little while. We'll let you know when we've finished." After the trauma they'd been through with Kaiser, the family appreciated St. Anne's Hospital's sensitivity and compassion.

I had remained behind at the mortuary. There were a lot of people there, and we had to tell them what had happened. I sat there in the pew, greeting everybody. Our bodies respond in mysterious ways, and I believe my level of shock is what kept me going.

The people who worked at the mortuary were kind and helpful. They went out and got coffee and cookies and pitched in to help us; they helped us through a difficult time.

I decided to go ahead with the rosary. Father McCarthy announced what happened so that I didn't have to explain it again, though we didn't know at that time that Lou had died. The priest included both Lou and Jenny in his prayers.

When the rosary was over, a close friend of mine took me to St. Anne's Hospital to join the rest of the family. We arrived at the hospital only to get the dreadful news that Lou was dead. I found that the rest of the family had already left the hospital to go back to the mortuary to give me the sad news. We had crossed paths on the road.

Our children were in total shock. I don't think any of them could shed any tears at that point. They returned to the mortuary, found people still standing outside, and told them of Lou's death. When Cathy told her uncle Nick what had happened, he couldn't believe it. "Oh, God!" he cried. His arms dropped, his knees buckled, and he lost his footing. Everyone thought he was going to drop. He and Lou had been very close.

That night we reflected on the day's events. We believe Lou chose to go with Jenny at that point. He left us at exactly the time when the whole family was there with him.

Amazing Grace had told him that Jenny wasn't going to suffer anymore, and that her daddy would never leave her. At her rosary, Lou kissed her and immediately joined her in Heaven. Grace was right. Jenny's daddy never left her.

9

Thou Art With Thine

Not till each loom is silent,
And the shuttles cease to fly,
Shall God reveal the pattern
And explain the reason why.
                                        Anonymous

Friday, March 7, 1986

The night Lou died, we somehow made it through Jenny's rosary. After we went to the hospital and found that Lou had not pulled through, our next step was breaking the news to our grandchildren at home. This was hard for us, since they were completely unaware of what had gone on all evening. Now we had to tell them their grandfather was dead.

I was so disoriented that night that I got out Lou's coat and started cleaning it so he could wear it at Jenny's burial service the next day. The house was full of people that evening, and we set up beds and cots everywhere. Cathy, Rosemarie and I all huddled in the same bed that night. We couldn't sleep. We shared the fear that one of us might be the next to die. In the days and months to come, the double tragedy exacted a heavy emotional and physical toll on each member of our family.

Rosemarie's suffering was intense. Ten minutes after the ambulance was called it had still not arrived, and a second call was made. She spent nearly 20 minutes giving Lou CPR chest compressions before the ambulance finally got there. Her arms were so sore that it took her two weeks to recover their full use. She was confined to the couch for days, and for two weeks she was too depressed to talk to anyone.

Cathy was working in Pacifica at the First National Bank of Daly City at the time. When Jenny died, the bank gave her three days off for the funeral. When she reported that her father had died during her sister's funeral, they gave her two entire months of compassionate leave.

Lou had been pronounced dead at St. Anne's Hospital in San Mateo County. Several days after Lou's funeral, Cathy and Vince drove to the coroner's office in San Mateo to pick up his belongings. On the way to the office, Cathy suffered a strong anxiety attack. It was as if the world were closing in on her. She felt as though her lungs wouldn't expand and that she couldn't breathe. The attack subsided by the time they got there, but both of them were unnerved when the clerk handed them Lou's wallet, his shoes, and his belt. The clothes evidently had been destroyed.

On the way back home, Cathy had another panic attack, and Vince took her to St. Anne's Hospital. There a nurse in the emergency room recognized her and ushered her in to see the doctor. He had been on call the night Lou had died and knew the stress she was under. Fortunately, she didn't require hospitalization, and Vince brought her home later that evening. Cathy was already under a great deal of stress at the time because of marital separation followed by divorce. Several sessions with a psychological counselor helped her cope with her anxiety.

As with the other family members, recovering from the double tragedy took years. "As painful as it is, grief is a natural process," Cathy says. "Although we all discussed the possibility of therapy to help us, none felt any special need for anything long-term. No matter what you do, recovering from the loss of a loved one is mostly a matter of time."

I was crushed by Lou's death. It all happened so suddenly that I never had the chance to tell him I loved him one last time.

That night I had a dream about Lou. He was sitting in our den, and he said to me, "Come over here and sit down by me, Dorothy. I have something to tell you."

I said, "No, I don't want to hear about it. It's all about Jenny, I know."

He said, "No," so I sat down next to him. He didn't say another word. He put his arms around my shoulders. I looked up, and on the coffee table in my dream there was a Bible. It was open, and a passage was underlined in red ink. The passage said, "*Thou art with thine.*"

I knew immediately what my dear husband had to say to me from beyond the grave: he and Jenny were reunited.

I was in complete shock for Jenny's funeral, as was Rosemarie. She sat in the second pew with a drained, blank look on her face. It was as though she was attending the funeral of a complete stranger. Her face was expressionless. That's how deep was the level of her shock.

I remember tears rolling down my eyes as I got into the limousine. "Well, here we go," I said to the children, for lack of something better to say. More than 100 friends and relatives attended Jenny's burial service.

That day was also Jenny's 30th birthday. Days before, when Lou and I had purchased the burial plots, we made arrangements with The New Southern, a local restaurant, to have food ready for the mourners who came long distances to attend the funeral. We also ordered a cake to honor Jenny's birthday.

When Lou died, we called the restaurant to cancel the arrangements. The family ate alone that day.

Saturday & Sunday, March 8–9, 1986

It had been a harrowing week, but we had work to do on Saturday. Cathy, Rosemarie and I returned to the mortuary and picked out Lou's casket and a suit to bury him in. We spent the rest of Saturday and Sunday resting at our respective homes.

Monday, March 10, 1986

On Monday, six days after Jenny died and three days after Lou died, Paulie left my home to live with his father, Paul. He had just turned eight. The day he left, Paulie said to me, "I'd like to stay with you, Nonie, but my Dad needs me, and I have to

another full year and a lawsuit before Kaiser would send us the full report.

When we finally read the autopsy report after waiting for so long, each of us reacted with such emotion that we thought we were reliving the day she died. There, in impersonal clinical detail was all the cold, hard, medical information about the condition of our daughter's body after the medical profession had finished with her.

The autopsy report described her as a "young Caucasian female 146 cm. in length with dark brown hair braided into two pigtails, gray-brown eyes, and permanent dentition in good repair." The condition of each major organ was described in detail, and a list was provided of the organs that were "surgically absent." The report concluded that Jenny died of "Acute Respiratory Distress Syndrome," the name for her condition at the time of death. But we knew that she died of medical negligence, which had led to the massive staph infection through her Hickman catheter, which led to infection of her lungs, pneumonia, lung collapse, two cardiac arrests, brain death, and final death.

December 25, 1986

On Christmas Day 1986, Cathy and I had a spiritual experience which gave us great comfort. We went to Holy Cross Cemetery to visit the graves that day.

Cathy recalls the scene: "As we walked in, we placed our flowers in the vases on the two crypts. As I raised up to put mine in Dad's vase, I heard and felt a deep, loud sound that startled me. It interrupted my prayers for Jenny and Dad. I was irritated. I said, 'Mom, what's that noise?' She heard it, too. The next thing we knew, we saw a whirlwind pick up leaves that had gathered in a corner and throw them in the air like a column. Then, as quickly as it appeared, it disappeared, and the noise went away. Mom and I looked at each other with tears in our eyes; we knew the spirits of Jenny and Dad were with us. We couldn't wait to get home to tell the family what we had just experienced."

After that point, we started telling Jenny's story to anyone who would listen.

10

Torture by Arbitration

> *No lesson seems to be so deeply inculcated*
> *by the experience of life as*
> *that you never should trust experts.*
> Lord Salisbury, 1877

> *You never expected justice from a company, did you?*
> *They neither have a soul to lose, nor a body to kick.*
> Sydney Smith, 1771-1845
> English writer and clergyman

To Sue or Not to Sue

Some time shortly after Jenny's death, a friend who knew her asked me if we were going to sue Kaiser for having caused Jenny's death. At the time, all we could think about was her loss. I told the friend that Jenny was dead, nothing could bring her back, and that we weren't interested in punishment, revenge, or profiting from her death. I was enraged at how Kaiser had treated Jenny and our family, but a lawsuit against Kaiser was just a legal action to which their legal staff would respond. Our pain was personal, but there was no way we could make them feel our pain. Corporations are abstract legal and financial entities, not flesh-and-blood people. They do not have hearts or souls, nerves or consciences. They are incapable of feeling pleasure or pain. At the time, we didn't see what good a lawsuit would do.

As time went on and the magnitude of Kaiser's malpractice became evident, our family started to see that a suit might produce some good from Jenny's tragedy. It might force Kaiser to release the autopsy report. It might expose Kaiser's callous treatment and professional incompetence.

The threat of having to pay damages might even force Kaiser to change the way they treated drug-dependent and chronically ill patients. Perhaps, we thought, if we sued, Kaiser might be forced to change their lethal ways. Maybe, just maybe, a suit could help assure that the next case like Jenny might be handled better.

After Jenny's death we were angry at Kaiser, but it took us a while to sort out the reasons why. As our grief subsided and our minds cleared, we were horrified when we mapped out what had happened to her there.

An HMO is a health care treatment pool. It is supposed to care for everyone according to their needs and spread the cost over all members. When Jenny became a Kaiser HMO member, she became entitled to all the rights and privileges available to any member. Many HMO members never require extreme or long-term forms of care; like Jenny, some do. Many never require frequent attention; like Jenny, some do. Some people can afford private medical insurance; some can't. Paul and Jenny knew both sides of that coin. When Paul's job qualified them for HMO coverage by Kaiser, his employer paid Kaiser's required insurance premiums for the family's medical care. As fully paid HMO members in good standing, Paul and Jenny had every right to expect that Jenny would receive appropriate medical care for whatever her problem might be. She didn't.

Jenny did not die a natural death, and Jenny did not die from natural causes. Kaiser's negligence and incompetence killed her.

The roots of Kaiser's malpractice went back to the first days of her treatment at Kaiser.

They viewed her long-term care needs as a financial liability to be minimized, not a problem to be solved. Therefore she got the cheapest care (home TPN), not the best or most appropriate care. They treated Jenny not as a patient in chronic pain, but as though she were a drug addict who was using Kaiser as her drug dealer. They dismissed her pain and treated her with contempt. They did everything they could to make her "just go away."

When she was delirious from her catheter infection, they dismissed it as problems with her painkiller dosages.

When she slipped and broke her hip in their hospital, they dismissed it as a bruise.

We asked for a gurney in advance when she couldn't walk with her broken hip; they ignored the request and put her in a wheelchair.

The doctors claimed to be ignorant of the puncture in her Hickman catheter, which was glaring proof that they did not consult her medical records when they treated her.

When three doctors dismissed her raging catheter infection as "the flu," they signed her death warrant.

Even when they suspected infection, they left the Hickman catheter in place. Had that been done to save the cost of replacing it?

After her death, when they left Jenny bloody and slumped half off the bed for us to see, they showed that they were incapable of even basic human respect and dignity.

And when they refused to release the final autopsy report or discuss it with the family, they showed us that all they wanted was to hide while they waited for us to go away.

Over the course of the year and a half that they treated Jenny, Kaiser's attitude toward her went from indifference to annoyance to aggravation to callousness and, finally, to contempt. The more she needed their expert diagnosis and care, the less willing they were to listen to her. They ignored her, scorned her, and mentally abused her for the entire time she was their patient.

By the time six months had passed after Jenny's and Lou's deaths, and our minds had cleared a bit, we started wondering several things. Reflecting on their unwillingness to release the autopsy report, our first and most obvious question was, "Why did Jenny die?"

Then, based on their unwillingness to talk to us, we asked ourselves, "What does Kaiser have to hide?"

Next, we looked at her care and asked, "Is Kaiser treating

other drug-dependent and chronically ill patients this way?"

Then we asked ourselves, "What can we do to make Kaiser change the way they treat patients like Jenny?"

Finally, we asked, "How can we help make sure that Kaiser improves the quality of their care so there will be no more cases like Jenny?"

We didn't want any other family to have to go through what our family did at Kaiser's hands. In the summer of 1986 we chose to file suit against Kaiser. Our first step was to find a qualified lawyer willing to take on the case.

The Lawyers

When we asked ourselves who should handle the case, we immediately thought of the famous San Francisco lawyer, Melvin Belli. We knew that we would be taking on one of the nation's largest and most powerful health care corporations, and we also knew that Mr. Belli had gone up against some of the nation's largest corporations before. We soon learned that California's limitation on malpractice damages made any damages from our case far too small to interest a lawyer of Mr. Belli's stature. His staff told us he wouldn't be able to consider our claim against Kaiser.

Some time before, when we realized that the Whipple procedure recommended by Dr. David had been radical beyond our wildest fears, a friend of Vince's had asked if we were going to sue. If so, the friend said, he knew about Elton Lazar, a San Rafael lawyer who specialized in wrongful death cases. The distinctive name stuck in Vince's memory. Years later, when we decided to sue Kaiser, we contacted Mr. Lazar and made an appointment.

Before visiting his office, we did what informed legal consumers are supposed to do. We called the California State Bar Association, and they said they had no record of any disciplinary actions against Mr. Lazar. This reassured us that we had made a good start, and we went to his office for the first meeting.

Mr. Lazar greeted us warmly, and we discussed the case. He seemed genuinely sympathetic and angry that Kaiser had treated Jenny and us so badly, and said his office could accept the case. He said that he handled general law cases, and that his colleague, Frank Hayes, specialized in malpractice. They would be working together, he said. Mr. Lazar seemed like a real go-getter, and Mr. Hayes seemed very pleasant.

After our meeting, the family got together and concluded that we liked Mr. Lazar and Mr. Hayes and that they seemed like the kind of men who were going to get in there and fight for us. I wrote a check for the $7,000 retainer required, and we all breathed a sigh of relief. Jenny's case was finally in good hands, we thought.

Several weeks into the case, the two lawyers invited the family to dinner to get to know us better and to discuss the case. Mr. Lazar told us that he was filing a multi-million dollar suit against Kaiser for the "negligent infliction of emotional distress" on behalf of the family as a result of Jenny's and Lou's deaths. Vince recalls, "We were impressed. Mr. Lazar convinced us that he felt our pain and knew what we were going through."

There were only two problems: under California law, "negligent infliction of emotional distress" is not permissible grounds for a civil suit. Furthermore, Kaiser's attorneys pointed out that they could not possibly be held responsible for Lou's death. He was not their patient, and they had never treated him. Our attorney had made two major blunders, resulting in a case that would be thrown out of any California court where it might be filed.

He compounded his bungling with procrastination. He asked Kaiser for a copy of the autopsy, and when it didn't arrive, he waited a full year before he sent a follow-up letter. He dragged his feet getting depositions from the Kaiser physicians, claiming, "Kaiser is being uncooperative." In California, you must get the case to trial within five years of filing suit. With the exception of taking depositions from our family members, which happened in September 1988, he did virtually nothing on the case for three years. Yes, three years.

Mr. Lazar never avoided our phone calls. He was always willing to talk with us, and each time we talked he assured us that everything was fine and that "these things take time." In fact, he was doing virtually nothing to move the case along. He evidently had given the case to Frank Hayes, but for reasons which were never explained, he and Hayes discontinued their working alliance, leaving the case back in Mr. Lazar's lap. This was a major problem, because it was now November 1990. The five-year statute of limitations would run out in March 1991, and our case was nowhere near ready to go to trial.

Mr. Lazar told us, "I'm trying to get a new lawyer." With only six months left before the statute of limitations ran out, we were in panic. He called a woman attorney he knew, and Rosemarie and I went to meet with her. At the end of the meeting, she said the case sounded solid and that she would confer with her partners.

The next day she called us and said, "You have a strong case, there's no doubt about it. But my firm and I are tied up with other cases already and we couldn't take on the work. There are depositions to be taken, exhibits to be prepared, and all within the next few months. We're too committed already. I'm sorry."

By then we were worried that all our efforts would come to nothing. Mr. Lazar's idea of a defense was to go to the judge on the appointed court day, plead that Kaiser had not been cooperative, throw the case on the mercy of the court, and pray that the judge would grant an extension. When Paul heard that, he called me and said, "He must be crazy!"

I called the other lawyer back and said, "We're in trouble here, and we need help. If you can't help us, can you give us the name of someone who can?"

She said, "Call Gary Moss, and tell him I told you to call." We got lucky. He took on the case. That, of course, required another $8,000 retainer. When we called, the California State Bar said that we might have grounds for a suit against Mr. Lazar, but we didn't have the time to file a complaint. We felt that Kaiser had killed Jenny. As her survivors, our priority was to see that she had her day in court.

Mr. Moss took over the case at a time when heroic efforts were required to save it from complete disaster. He proved to be the right man for the job.

After reviewing the evidence, he filed suit on behalf of Paul and Paulie Gigliello against Kaiser Foundation Health Plan, Inc., for $250,000 (the maximum allowable under California law) for the wrongful death of their wife and mother.

The Arbitration

Kaiser immediately demanded that the suit be settled by arbitration. This clause was part of their contract with all Kaiser HMO members, so there was no alternative. Early in 1992, Mr. Moss took the depositions from the physicians who treated Jenny at Kaiser (the work that our previous lawyer should have done four years earlier).

Early on, Mr. Moss asked us whether we wanted a quick settlement or a full arbitration. In a conversation with Rosemarie, he suggested that Kaiser would probably be willing to settle out of court for $50,000 or $75,000 if we asked for it. We told him no. We weren't interested in the money. We wanted Kaiser's treatment of Jenny to be publicly explored and put on the record. We wanted everything out in the open for everyone to see. We weren't looking for a quick settlement. We said, "Thank you, Gary, but that's not what we want. This is all for Jenny. Let's see it through to the end."

No matter what happened, Kaiser stood to lose no more than $250,000 if they were found liable for Jenny's death. We were not looking for the money, but we felt strongly that if they didn't have to pay financially for her death, there would be little incentive for them to change their ways.

The $250,000 cap on malpractice liability was instituted as one method to reduce the enormous cost of malpractice insurance. Years of multi-million dollar legal judgments for "pain and suffering" had driven up the cost of liability insurance for doctors to over $100,000 per year. This, in turn, was passed along to medical consumers in the form of higher prices for health care. The $250,000 cap on the amount any plaintiff could receive in a malpractice suit proved to be helpful in limiting the rate at which the cost of health care grows, but at the same time, it took away a powerful tool to force medical practitioners to practice their medicine responsibly.

The case would be heard by an arbitration judge and two arbitrators, one appointed by Kaiser and one by our attorneys. The proceedings took place in a building in Oakland that housed Kaiser's attorneys. The arbitration took place in a conference room, not a courtroom. The neutral arbitrator was the Honorable Winston Holmes, a retired judge. Kaiser had their arbitrator and attorneys; we had ours. The only other people present were the court reporter and the witnesses.

The arbitration dragged on over three years, from 1992 to 1995 because the proceedings frequently were adjourned and postponed. Getting the attorneys and witnesses all together in one room was forever a problem, and a death in a family or a conflict with another case always seemed to conspire to make it impossible for the arbitration board to meet. Rosemarie, Paul and I went to the first arbitration hearing, which lasted for several days. The room was small, so only those directly involved and who had given depositions could attend. That excluded Cathy and Vince.

At that first meeting we heard a statement from the neutral arbitrator which we would hear again and again: "Ladies and gentlemen, we haven't finished with this witness today, but he has to be in surgery (or in court, or out of town) tomorrow, so we're going to have to find another day when we can all get together again. I'm adjourning the proceeding for now. Attorneys will please make appropriate arrangements for the next session. Adjourned."

It usually took two or three months (sometimes more) to get together again, and then they only got a day or two of work done before adjourning again. This went on for three years.

It was extremely frustrating for us. We had given our depositions three years earlier, and now it was time to tell the story once and for all in front of the arbitrators. Yet when we were ready to take the stand, there was always some delay. It was maddening. It seemed as if we would never get the weight of the proceeding off our shoulders.

Rosemarie probably suffered more than anyone. She was the main witness to Jenny's condition, and she was closest to Jenny's care in the last two years. She remembers being shocked at the casualness of the whole proceeding. It was our daughter and sister who had died, and between witnesses, the arbitrators and lawyers were discussing their private lives.

To us, it seemed almost as bad as at Kaiser; no respect for the dead. They talked about the private schools their kids were attending and the Arabian horses they were training. It was pretty clear that they didn't care much about the subject they were litigating. The arbitrators and the attorneys were all very chummy, as they discussed their plans for the weekend. It was very disconcerting for our family, who took these proceedings very seriously.

Kaiser had all the advantages in this case. They were the rich HMO, and they could hire all the expert witnesses they wanted. They hired eight people to testify for them. We only had two. But ours were the best: Dr. Ronald Estil and Dr. Mason Farmer.

Rosemarie was angered by the lies that were told on the record by Kaiser staff people. She was particularly incensed when Dr. Barber refused to acknowledge that his conference with her or his promise to discuss the final autopsy report with the family ever took place.

We were appalled that the emergency room physicians who examined Jenny when she was delirious, alleged that they told her and the family that she was very sick and should be admitted to the hospital. This was an outright lie, of course, and there was no mention of this in the records they wrote. They were obviously covering up. I remember sitting there in the room as they told one untruth after another. I could hear my heart beating, it affected me so.

We attended every arbitration session. We listened to every expert witness for each side. Every Kaiser witness said basically the same thing: Kaiser met the minimum "standard of care" for every one of Jenny's medical problems.

Our expert witnesses refuted that. In each case, they showed beyond any possible doubt that Kaiser had inadequate plans, inadequate staff training, inadequate supervision, and exercised bad judgment to boot.

It was hard for me to listen to the Kaiser witnesses repeating "We met the standards of care" like so many trained parrots. Every time I heard that I would cringe and have to look up at the ceiling to keep the tears in my eyes from flowing. That was my dead daughter they were talking about, who died from their "standards of care." A number of times I couldn't take it any longer and left the room to regain my composure. I didn't want to break down in the arbitration room.

Scheduled meetings often were canceled on short notice or no notice at all. This happened three or four times. We had to make special preparations to attend, so it was hard on everyone. I lived in Rohnert Park by this time, which is an hour and a half drive from Oakland, and Rosemarie lived in Novato. We would make our transportation plans, coordinate them with Paul Sr., show up, and often find that the arbitration meeting was canceled.

The proceeding dragged on so long and in so many disconnected segments that the lawyers on both sides prepared extensive, two-pound closing briefs to bring the judge and the arbitrators up-to-date on the whole proceeding.

The night before the final arbitration hearing, when the closing arguments were to be given, I got a call from Gary Moss, reminding us to be there on time.

"Are you ready to go?" he asked.

"We sure are," I replied.

"I just wanted to make sure you knew it was tomorrow," he told me.

"I wouldn't miss it for anything," I assured him. "Rosemarie, Paul and I will be there." It had been five months since the last hearing. We knew this was going to be it (the big one). The last stand. The final testimony to vindicate Jenny. We wouldn't have missed it for the world.

The next morning at nine o'clock sharp, we arrived at the arbitration hearing office. "There is no arbitration today," a clerk informed us.

Rosemarie was outraged. She had to arrange to take unpaid leave from work to be at these hearings. "What do you mean there is no arbitration today?" she fumed.

"There was a death in the family of one of the arbitrators," the woman replied.

"A death?" Rosemarie asked.

"Well, a memorial service."

Someone had chosen to go to a memorial service rather than proceed with the case. We should have known. But we didn't. Here we thought we saw the end of the tunnel, and they had canceled the proceeding. We were angry. Nobody cared.

The arbitrators decided to hand in their closing briefs and let it go at that. No final statements. The arbitration was over. We were waiting for our arbitrator to lay out Kaiser's callousness and incompetence in a nice, neat presentation, point by point. We wanted to hear it. When they folded their cards and handed in the briefs without any verbal presentation, it was a huge emotional letdown for us.

The Ruling

On February 10, 1995, nine years after Jenny's death, and four years after Gary Moss took over the case, the arbitrators finally rendered their ruling. I learned about the settlement over the phone from Gary. "We won the case," he said.

The most the arbitrators could have awarded was $250,000. The arbitrators held Kaiser wholly responsible for Jenny's premature death. Their judgment for $175,000 rather than the full $250,000 was based upon their assumption that Jenny, 29 at the time of her death, would only have lived three to ten years longer in any case. In his deposition, Dr. Barber estimated five years. That piece of information stunned us. Until that time, no one had ever suggested to us that Jenny's life expectancy had been shortened by the medical madness. Both Dr. David and Dr. Barber talked to us about Jenny living a long, normal life. Maybe we should have known better, but the fact was never brought to our attention.

$65,218.25 went to the lawyers and to the costs of arbitration. Paul and Paul, Jr. received $82,281 as compensation for the loss of their wife and mother. $3,500 was distributed to Paul, Jr. immediately so that he could buy a car to use for work. His remaining share was deposited in a bank until he reached the age of 18. The money is designated for his education. The balance of the award was paid to his father, Paul Sr.

It was a clear-cut decision and a moral victory. The process left us triumphant but exhausted. The arbitrators agreed that Kaiser was solely responsible for Jennifer's death.

11

No More Jennys

Cur'd yesterday of my disease,
I died last night of my physician.
Matthew Prior, 18th century English poet

Prevention

After the arbitration panel finally agreed that Kaiser's negligence caused Jenny's death, we tried to get on with our lives, yet none of us felt any closure from the panel's decision. In talking to each other, we all found that we were wondering the same things. All over the country, patients were being crippled, maimed, and killed by well-known doctors and HMOs with good reputations. We asked ourselves how future tragedies like Jenny's could be prevented. What can patients and their families do to ensure that their loved ones receive good, safe medical care when a doctor says they need an operation? How can patients ensure they will be treated humanely, safely, and competently when they enter an HMO hospital for care?

To understand what needed to be changed, we went back and analyzed each step of Jenny's medical history. We found that serious, preventable errors were made at almost every stage of her treatment.

We saw that our biggest mistake was to trust what we were told and not ask questions. We now realize that the patient must take a far more active role in making major health decisions than Jenny and our family took. We now know that by relying solely on the physicians, we permitted decisions to be made and actions to be taken that we would never permit now. At crucial junctures in Jenny's care, we didn't have enough information to make informed choices.

Jenny's long slide from vigorous health to lingering death took place in two stages. In the first, incompetent private physicians turned her into a partially disabled person who was dependent upon narcotic painkillers. In the second stage, Kaiser's obsession to maximize profits prolonged her excruciating pain. Soon thereafter, their incompetence killed her. Here are the problems we confronted, followed by some conclusions that might help others.

The Beginning

When Jenny had her first severe pain attack while she was pregnant, she wrote it off as a fluke and failed to tell her gynecologist or any other physician about it. The attack was never evaluated, so the opportunity to learn anything was lost.

Her second attack, six weeks after Paulie was born, was serious. She was doubled up in agony and vomited green bile. The physicians at the Bayview Hospital emergency room examined her thoroughly, but didn't find the source of the pain and sent her home. This second attack should have alerted her and us that something significant was wrong. Jenny was covered by private health insurance at the time. Had the Bayview physicians recommended that she see a specialist, or had Jenny done so on her own, a diagnosis might have been reached.

When the third attack struck, Paul took Jenny to Dr. Barbara Thomas, who recognized the seriousness and rushed her to Mt. Hope Hospital. This was the first good thing that happened in her care. At the hospital, gastroenterologist Dr. Alfred Ellis believed that her gallbladder was causing her problems and recommended that it be removed. My husband and I both thought that Jenny was too young to need a gallbladder operation, so we asked for a second opinion. A physician friend recommended Dr. Eric R. David, a surgeon.

Dr. David

Dr. David felt the problem was an inflamed pancreas, and recommended against the gallbladder removal. In retrospect, this was a critical juncture. The decision to trust Dr. David led to Jenny's slide into a life full of pain. Getting a second opinion before permitting Jenny to undergo an operation was a good decision. Choosing Dr. David turned out to be a very bad one.

Based on the medical evidence revealed during the arbitration process, we now believe that Jenny's acute relapsing pancreatitis was caused by gallstones. Her symptoms fit a diagnosis of gallstone pancreatitis; they did not fit pancreatitis caused by any other common factor.

In adults, the gallbladder can be removed with virtually no adverse effect on the patient. The operation is simple and low-risk. We now believe that if Jenny's gallbladder had been removed in late 1978, her problems probably would have disappeared with it. It would no longer produce gallstones to pass through her system and lodge in her pancreas. Without irritation, inflammation of the pancreas would not have continued.

Problems Escalate

In retrospect, a number of problems are evident to us at this stage in Jenny's care. First, was our lack of sufficient information about Jenny's condition. We didn't know the different causes of pancreatitis. We didn't know the difference between the pain caused by gallstones and the pain caused by pancreatic inflammations.

Second, we assumed that all doctors were equally good, and we chose to listen to the advice of Dr. David. We never stopped to think that a doctor's judgment might be affected by concerns other than his patient's health.

Third, as Jenny's pain attacks increased in frequency and duration and were accompanied by vomiting and malnutrition, she did not go back to consult with her primary care physician. Instead, she relied on emergency room physicians and Dr. David.

Fourth, our ignorance about Dr. David's qualifications kept us from realizing that we were not getting our information from the best-qualified source. Emergency room physicians only have the responsibility to examine a patient, stabilize their condition, and refer them to a specialist. They made no referral, and Jenny evidently felt that Dr. David was her specialist. He wasn't. He was a general surgeon. He had no specialized knowledge of pancreatic diseases. Dr. David never volunteered that information, and we didn't have enough medical knowledge to determine it ourselves.

Finally, Jenny should have requested an examination by a pancreas specialist. Because we assumed that Dr. David knew everything he needed to know about the procedures he recommended, it never dawned on us or Jenny to ask for a specialist's opinion.

At this point Dr. David recommended "a pancreas operation." He told the family little except that it should help. The pancreatic duct drainage he performed in 1980 revealed a stone. Jenny's attacks continued, however, and now she could no longer hold down solid food.

Jenny's health care took a major turn for the worse at this time. She became emaciated.

She was experiencing a crisis, and if something wasn't done, she would die of malnutrition at the age of 22. Did Dr. David press hard to discover the real cause of the pain attacks and the vomiting? No. In conjunction with physicians at Memorial Hospital, he decided to treat the symptom of the disease (malnutrition) rather than the disease itself. His course of action: surgically implant a Hickman catheter into her body, and feed her through the catheter.

Placement of the Hickman catheter (a high-risk device at best) further strained her already-weakened body and added an entire new layer of risk. Now Jenny had two threats to her life to deal with: her original condition, still undiagnosed, and the Hickman catheter. This crucial mistake completely ignored the still-undiagnosed source of her pain and vomiting and permitted her condition to deteriorate.

Why did no one go after the root cause of Jenny's problem? Only Dr. David knows. By this time, he was the only physician with anything like a comprehensive picture of Jenny's medical condition. Why didn't Jenny or our family insist on finding the root cause? Because when her doctor said it was the pancreas, we believed him.

Two years after the initial pain attack, the cause was still undiagnosed, and the pain continued to strike. Now Dr. David recommended that he perform the Whipple Procedure on Jenny. Again, he told Jenny and the family little about the operation, saying only "it would help." He opened her up, performed the surgery and found a stone in her pancreatic duct, but left out one of the standard steps: he failed to remove the gallbladder.

Why didn't Jenny or the family ask for a second opinion before permitting the operation? We continued to trust the doctor, not knowing he was withholding from all of us the complexity, scope, and risk of the operation. Jenny and our family, like most people, had no specialized medical education. We had no knowledge that the Whipple was normally only used in advanced cases of pancreatic cancer.

Now we know what we didn't know then (but what Dr. David surely must have known): Jenny's pancreas problems could have been remedied with a partial pancreatectomy, a relatively uncomplicated operation for removal of part of the pancreas. Instead, he chose the invasive, high-risk Whipple Procedure.

Why did Dr. David withhold the risk information from us, ignore the risks, and perform the Whipple anyway? We'll never know. In doing so, he appears to have overlooked the first obligation required by the Hippocratic Oath; that is, do no harm. He also ignored a cardinal rule of medicine: always choose the course of action that offers the best chance of success and the least risk to the patient. He did the opposite.

After the operation, the pain continued, and new problems stemming from the Whipple procedure dwarfed Jenny's original problem. Since all but the tail of her pancreas had been surgically removed, where could the pain be coming from? She still had her gallbladder.

Now, without pancrease being produced by her pancreas, she couldn't digest solid foods. In addition, Dr. David had removed part of her digestive tract during the Whipple, and now her food raced through her system before it could be absorbed. Thus, malnutrition became a continual and irreversible problem. Still no one sought to find the original source of the pain that continued to plague her.

More Doctors, More Surgeries

On April 1, 1983, Dr. David performed another operation on Jenny's intestinal tract. The pain did not disappear. The persistence of her pain led to progressively larger doses of painkillers; she became dependent on Demerol for relief of that pain.

Dr. Hobson became involved in trying to minimize her use of the painkillers and help her avoid drug dependence, but with Jenny's move from San Francisco to Novato, he was too far away to continue to treat her.

On May 10, 1984, Dr. Allen G. Stokes performed Jenny's final pancreatic surgery. This removed the last portion of her pancreas, leaving her an insulin-dependent diabetic. Dr. Stokes also saw the evidence of the previous surgeries by Dr. David. The physicians' code of silence (and possible concerns of a libel suit) evidently kept Dr. Stokes from telling Jenny and the family about what he saw.

Kaiser Problems Begin

We kept going back to the gallbladder as the possible root of the problem, and Dr. Stokes wrote to Dr. Barber at Kaiser suggesting that the gallbladder be removed. Jenny and the family never saw the report. Dr. Barber evidently didn't agree with it. Why did he disagree with the specialist? We will never know. Jenny's gallbladder stayed in. Her pain increased.

When Paul Gigliello took a job with a firm providing HMO health care through the Kaiser Foundation Hospital, Jenny felt as though someone was again watching out for her health. She was wrong. Kaiser quickly stopped treating her as a patient in need of a cure, and started treating her as a financial liability they hoped would go away. This was a major problem for Jenny, for she was dependent on Kaiser's staff for her very life. She had only one place to go for her care, so she didn't dare make Kaiser mad.

When she became a Kaiser patient, Jenny had been off TPN for a year. When Kaiser reinstated the TPN, they not only had her use it for nutrients but, as a cost-cutting measure, they also had her perform the far more critical procedure of injecting her painkiller and her insulin into the Hickman. This required a complex flushing procedure every three hours every day. As Paul states, "That was over our heads." Jenny still was wracked with pain and malnutrition and made trip after trip to the hospital. Kaiser provided a home health care nurse to check her, but the twice-weekly visits were inadequate to the challenge.

Other hospitals had achieved excellent records with home

TPN, but Kaiser evidently never studied their programs. Jenny was the first home TPN patient at Kaiser, San Rafael. She became their guinea pig. Kaiser's home TPN program was a farce. Their staff was untrained, and their safety procedures existed only on paper.

Nationwide, HMOs are under constant fire for their failure to call in specialists on complicated cases like Jenny's. The reason they don't is simple: specialists cost money and cut into profits. Although her condition was deteriorating before their eyes, Kaiser never referred Jenny to a pancreas specialist.

We knew nothing about the fatal flaw at Kaiser that triggered Jenny's death spiral until it was too late.

Dr. Henry Barber, who had been supervising her care at Kaiser, left on vacation without ensuring that special instructions were left in her records. Emergency Room staff personnel were untrained in diagnosing catheter infections. When Jenny started showing all the classic symptoms of a severe catheter infection, the examining physicians both dismissed it as the flu. Dr. Barber's backup was never consulted. By the time the error was discovered, Jenny's infection was far past the point of no return. She was doomed.

Problem: At Kaiser, no one physician was in charge of Jenny's care.

No physician had overall responsibility or accountability for knowing everything that happened to Jenny, knowing who treated her with what, planning her care, and getting her the specialist she needed. Most of her care and treatment was given by whichever emergency room physician was on duty. That doctor had no knowledge of her case except from what was written in her patient records. And, as we have seen, those records were often three to seven days out of date.

In recent years, HMOs have largely adopted the practice of appointing a primary care physician to oversee everything that happens to a patient. If this policy had been in effect at Kaiser when Jenny was there, her suffering and death might have been avoided or postponed.

Problem: Kaiser's staff treated Jenny in a callous, unprofessional, and inhumane manner.

Poor staff attitudes and unprofessional behavior can exist

only if the HMO's management tolerates them. Kaiser was negligent in failing to detect and eliminate these problems through sensitivity training and corrective counseling. HMOs typically cite the added costs of such training as the reason it is impossible to provide it. However, that response is usually a smokescreen to disguise a lack of willingness to acknowledge that problems exist and need to be solved.

Patients who experience poor treatment must take the initiative and demand better treatment. Defensive documentation is a powerful tool. Patients should carefully and openly record the names, dates, places and details of any rude, unprofessional, or negligent treatment they receive from their caregivers. Next, they should provide supervisors, physicians, or hospital management with written complaints and demand that the complaints be answered. If the standard of care does not improve, the patient should escalate the complaints by going to higher and higher levels in the hospital/HMO chain of command. If the conditions are serious, these detailed written records will prove invaluable if the problem must be taken to a state or federal regulatory agency or to court.

Problem: HMOs have no incentive to give good care to the chronically ill.

For HMOs, it is cheaper to let chronically ill patients die than to take care of them. Jenny's premiums at Kaiser were $55 per month; she was costing Kaiser thousands of dollars a month in care. HMOs have become profitable by treating short-term illnesses. By the time she became involved with Kaiser, Jenny needed almost continuous care, and for the conditions she had, she was going to require care for the rest of her life. Because of her surgeries, she often became malnourished. This would require hospitalization to build her up again. Kaiser did some fast arithmetic and saw that she was going to be a major financial drain on them if the repeated hospitalizations continued.

Even when Jenny's problems multiplied, and the use of painkillers and insulin became part of her daily routine, Kaiser kept her on home TPN so she could be treated as an outpatient. During the arbitration process Kaiser frequently said, "We gave her adequate care." They did not give her the best care, because it was expensive. They took the chance that the cheap way would be good enough, and they knew that if she died, their malpractice liability would be limited by California law to a maximum of $250,000. It was much cheaper for Kaiser to take the chance that she would die than to keep caring for her for another 10 to 20 years. And that is exactly what happened.

Problem: Patients with chronic illness are sometimes blamed for their condition.

When a family or their caregivers are dealing with a chronically ill patient, they face a frustrating task. They want the patient to get better, but when he or she doesn't get better, even they sometimes start blaming the patient, rather than the medical condition, for their problems. They think, "Well, if the doctors can't find the problem, maybe there isn't a problem. Maybe it's all in the patient's head." Only education and compassion can overcome this flawed perspective.

Problem: Patients in chronic pain are often treated like common drug addicts.

By the time Jenny had undergone the Whipple procedure at the age of 24, she was in constant pain. She could not carry on the normal duties of a wife and mother without the frequent use of powerful painkillers. As with thousands of other chronically ill patients, and through no fault of her own, she became dependent upon these prescribed medicines. As soon as that happened, Kaiser started treating her like a common drug addict.

As her pain continued, one might have expected understanding and sympathy from the health care professionals who had come to know her and her predicament. Jenny got the opposite. Kaiser's staff showed callous and inexcusable indifference to her plight. Instead of receiving compassionate care, she was constantly forced to prove that she was in sufficient pain to warrant the painkillers.

Before her move to Novato, Dr. David implied that Jenny might be demanding more painkillers than she really needed, but when pressed for evidence of this, he admitted that he had no way of determining her minimum needs. At Kaiser, this implication was repeated so often that after a while, both Jenny and our family started wondering if it might be true. There is something drastically wrong with a medical care system that places the blame for a patient's pain on the patient instead of on the illness.

Jenny was required to be examined by a psychiatrist to determine whether she was actually in severe pain or faking it to get drugs. Again, the burden of proof was on her. She had to satisfy the doctor that she was coming to the hospital because of real pain, not because she wanted a fix for her addiction.

When famous alcohol or drug addicts like former First Lady Betty Ford and movie star Elizabeth Taylor sought help for their addictions, they received compassionate care and were praised for seeking help. Jenny didn't fare as well. As she became a familiar face around the hospital, the Kaiser staff started to regard her as a nuisance and treat her as a burden instead of a patient in severe pain.

Because of the American government's war on illegal drugs, physicians who prescribe large or long-term doses of addictive drugs are closely scrutinized. This scrutiny generally works in the best interests of society, but may have an adverse effect on the welfare of the chronically ill, who often require progressively greater amounts of painkillers to deal with their increasing tolerance for the drugs.

A special medical treatment classification is needed for the many patients like Jenny who are dependent upon narcotic painkillers for their chronic pain. If this were done, they could receive the levels of painkillers they need to carry on their lives without suffering the indignity of discrimination. In addition, the physicians treating them would be removed from the unnecessary scrutiny that inhibits some from giving their chronically ill patients the painkillers they desperately need.

Furthermore, medical staff who deal with the chronically ill need better training about the special needs of these patients. They also need sensitivity training to keep them from exhibiting the callousness that permeated Kaiser's treatment of Jenny. Unfortunately, training that increases the quality of patient care costs money and reduces HMO profits. In the profit-oriented world of American HMOs, this educational funding is difficult to find.

Problem: Incompetent treatment is too often tolerated by the medical community.

Jenny's experience clearly demonstrated that, in California, if an HMO kills someone through malpractice, the HMO has little to fear. Although the arbitrators found Kaiser liable for Jenny's wrongful death, the Kaiser physicians who were responsible were never reprimanded, punished, or suspended. Their professional lives went on unchanged.

In Jenny's case, neither Kaiser nor its emergency room procedures were investigated as a result of our lawsuit. The litigation bothered them about as much as a cow flicking a fly off its back.

Since California law limits wrongful death judgments to a maximum of $250,000 and this sum is small by HMO standards, it poses no threat whatsoever. For this reason, HMOs are under little pressure to change practices that result in the death of their patients. Further, many private attorneys will no longer accept wrongful death cases, because they know law limits their monetary reward.

Had it not been for Kaiser's incompetence, Jenny would have been able to live many years beyond her 30th birthday, instead of dying of a massive undiagnosed staph infection. At Kaiser, under-trained physicians made grossly bad judgment calls. No one ever shut down their home TPN program so the staff could be trained to properly care for their surviving TPN patients.

Incompetent doctors need to be punished and retrained. HMOs must be required to submit their defective procedures to outside review. In specialties where they have been shown to be incompetent, HMOs should not be permitted to practice these until they are recertified.

Problem: Patients and their families often lack strong patient advocates.

The Hippocratic Oath alone no longer governs how health care is delivered in the United States. In HMOs, profit-seeking accountants increasingly make life-or-death decisions rather than doctors. Because of this, today's patients need someone in their corner, looking out for their rights. This person is the patient advocate.

Whether it is the patient himself, a member of the family, or a trusted friend, every seriously ill patient needs an advocate to get him the information and treatment he needs. In case the patient cannot get the information about their illness, treatment options, and possible threats to the quality of their life, a knowledgeable advocate needs to be available to stand up for the patient and his rights.

Patients who are about to enter a hospital for a serious medical problem should select a relative, close friend, or private nurse as their patient advocate before they are admitted. This would help assure that they had someone to push for information and explore treatment options, in case a patient's capacity to do it for himself is diminished by his medical condition.

The patient advocate should be a person with a broad knowledge of medicine and the health care system. She or he needs to be calm, assertive, and a very good listener, for it is the advocate's role to help make sure that doctors and hospitals hear and understand what the patient feels it is important to tell them. Likewise, the advocate must be perceptive enough to determine when the patient or family members have misconstrued information given to them by health care providers. Patient advocacy might well become an important new specialty within the nursing profession.

Had Jenny had a patient advocate to talk with about the Whipple procedure, she never would have gone under Dr. David's knife, and she would have been spared the years of agony she endured. Had Jenny had a patient advocate when she went to Kaiser's emergency room in a delirious state, the advocate could have insisted that she not be discharged until the true cause of the delirium had been established.

Had all these things happened, Jenny might well be alive today.

Patients Need Knowledge

In these days of corporate medicine and managed care, patients must persistently press for answers to their health care questions until they get them. Patients must also become experts in the care and treatment of their own diseases.

Knowledge is the key to beating life-threatening illnesses. In the mid-1980s when Jenny was in the midst of her traumatic experiences, medical information was not nearly as available as it is today. Access to most of the best medical information was restricted to doctors and health care professionals. In the last decade, the availability of high-quality medical information has increased immensely. The sources now include:

• Primary care physicians and other directly involved medical staff. These health care professionals are closest to the situation and can provide valuable insights not available from medical journals and databases. However they are often strapped for time, and they may not have the communication skills or personalities to match their medical expertise. Patients may have to approach them several times and use different approaches, in order to get the information they need.

• Libraries. In most public libraries today, one may find high-quality reference materials on almost any medical condition, course of treatment or therapy. If more information is needed, the reference librarian can usually obtain the needed materials on inter-library loan or refer the patron to an appropriate medical library.

• The Internet. The widespread availability of cheap Internet access has revolutionized access to medical information. For example, a thirty-second Internet search for information on "prostate cancer" located more than 500 reports, studies and papers that are immediately available for reading, downloading, or printing. A similar search for "pancreatitis" located more than 50 documents. In addition, hundreds of Internet "newsgroups" (public forums) exist to give people with a specific concern the ability to meet and discuss therapies and cures. For those people without personal computers equipped to access the Internet, many public libraries provide public access computer terminals.

Armed with accurate, up-to-date information on their problem, patients are in a good position to actively question their health care providers about their condition and the options available. As Jenny's husband, Paul, said several months after the arbitration was over, "If we had known more about her condition and options, we would have pressed Kaiser for better care."

On the Internet, the Johns Hopkins Medical Institutions Information Network (InfoNet) lists more than 250 phone numbers (many of them tollfree) on more than 100 topics that deal with patient advocacy questions; they cover everything from adoption to xeroderma pigmentosa. They also list nearly 200 web sites, with links to those sites. At the time of this book's publication, the Internet address for this listing was http://infonet.welch.jhu.edu/advocacy.html. InfoNet also directs the inquirer to other advocacy contacts, such as Med Help International (http://medhelp.org/search) and California Nurses Association (CNA) (http://www.califnurses.org/can/search). At the time of this writing, the CNA site published a "Kaiser Casualty of the Day" page as part of their Patient Watch program, in which they publicize "the human cost of corporate healthcare."

The National Organization of Physicians Who Care (http://www.pwc.org/index.html), organized in 1985 and head-quartered in San Antonio, Texas, claims a membership of 30,000 physicians who seek HMO reforms. A recent news article on their web site was titled, "HMO Patients Need to Ask Questions." They also provide a form to send e-mail to congress, and they sponsor the HMO Homepage on the Internet (http://www.hmopage.org), which lists a tollfree HMO hotline phone number for complaints.

Epilogue

The most frustrating part of this ordeal has been that Jenny's death did not bring about any changes at Kaiser. This huge HMO system appears to continue the same policies, including cutting back on patient care, that it followed in 1986. In 1997 it was reported that the State of Texas was considering revoking Kaiser's license to practice medicine. State officials there claimed that the large number of wrongful death lawsuits brought against Kaiser shows that Kaiser has been endangering patients' lives through excessive cost-cutting. The California Nurses Association continues to document such cases.

As for the Kaiser doctors responsible for Jenny's death, all are either still practicing at Kaiser, have voluntarily moved into private practice or have retired.

All of our family members take their health and health care much more seriously now than we did a decade ago. If one gets sick, the others all pay close attention. We take better care of ourselves, and we look out for each other. We don't rely on doctors to make all our medical decisions anymore. Jenny's mistreatment and death is still very much on our minds, and we spend more time together as a family, knowing now how precious that time is.

In 1996, our family got involved with promoting the passage of California Proposition 216, the Patient Protection Act. The legislation, which was supported by the California Nurses

Association, was designed to right many of the wrongs which led to Jenny's death. Among other things, it would have banned bonuses and financial incentives which encourage health care providers to deny patient care. It would have required a second opinion by a doctor who has examined a patient before critical care can be denied. It would have prohibited "gag orders" on doctors and nurses which prevent them from disclosing treatment options not covered by the insurer. Finally, it would have prohibited HMO's from forcing patients to agree to mandatory binding arbitration as a condition of health coverage.

I donated the postage, and my daughter, Cathy, and I and spent days stuffing envelopes with brochures, and mailing them to doctors on behalf of this legislation. After massive, well-financed opposition from the HMOs and the insurance industry, the proposition narrowly lost at the polls in November, 1996.

A March, 1999 column by Tom Abate in the San Francisco Chronicle reported on a lawsuit being filed, alleging that Kaiser was "... forcing doctors to cut costs at the same time it was spending $60 million a year to attract new members with ads claiming that doctors, not administrators, were in charge of care."

It is relatively easy to document the need for effective patient-fights legislation; the hard part is overcoming the special interests and their legislative servants who continue to prevent it.

Appendix A

A Letter from Amazing Grace

In the years after Jenny's death, we often wondered if Amazing Grace, the psychic who blessed Lou's handkerchief, had any knowledge of what had happened, or why. We always hoped we would be able to talk to her, but she evidently did not return to California. In 1997, Cathy made a search of the World Wide Web and found that Grace now had a home page there.

On March 3, 1997, the 11th anniversary of Jenny's death, Cathy wrote to Grace, telling her about our experience and asking about that night and the blessing. The next day, Grace replied by e-mail.

From: ~ Grace~<aerogirl@bestweb.net>
Subject: Re: Palace of fine arts in 1986
Dear Cathy,

I am glad that you have written to me after all these years by finding our web site. Of course I will pray for the soul of your father and your sister. I am sure they are not only at peace but in fact since they are with our Lord and Savior Jesus Christ. They are in fact praying to him for you and for the family that they left behind. That YOU all have the peace that surpasses understanding! Perhaps this is how you found the web site.

I am afraid that I do not have any concrete answers to your question as to what I felt or what I knew. When the Lord chooses to use me, and I am under His precious anointing. I am not always aware of the hows or whys of what He is directing me to do—but He is.

I am very glad for your sister that the Lord gave me a word of knowledge, that she would never be suffering again, and that, in fact, she would be with him shortly, and also for the direction the Lord left me with for your father.

I believe that your father felt the Holy Presence of the Lord that night and that his heart was being prepared for what was about to come, that he himself would be going home to be with the Lord. I believe that the Lord was blessing him with a preview of His mighty and unconditional love, and letting him know just how special and loved that he was.

I pray dear friend that you have peace in the knowledge that your precious relatives are now with Our Savior, and that in time you will be with them for all eternity.

God Bless You,
In Jesus' Love,
Grace

Appendix B

Further Information

The National Pancreas Foundation: To support the research of diseases of the pancreas, and to provide information and humanitarian services to those people who are suffering from such illness. A nonprofit organization, the NPF was founded by two families whose lives have been forever changed by the devastation of pancreatic cancer and chronic pancreatitis. The National Pancreas Foundation, P.O. Box 600590, Newtonville, MA 02460, Tel 1-877-NPF-FUND, http://trfn.clpgh.org/npf/

The American Pain Society: This is a multidisciplinary educational and scientific organization dedicated to serving people in pain. The society was founded in 1978 as a national chapter of the International Association for the Study of Pain, and now includes more than 3,200 physicians, nurses, psychologists, dentists, scientists, pharmacologists, therapists and social workers who research and treat pain and advocate for patients with pain. American Pain Society, 4700 W. Lake Avenue, Glenview, IL 60025, Tel 847-375-4715, www.ampainsoc.org/

Be Informed: Questions To Ask Your Doctor Before You Have Surgery. Learning more about your operation will help you make better decisions about your health care. U.S. Department of Health and Human Services, Executive Office Center Suite 501, 2101 East Jefferson Street, Rockville, MD 20252, www.pueblo.gsa.gov/cic_text/health/surgryqa/surgryqa.htm

Getting a Second Opinion: A full page of very informative information. www.1-a-market.com/health/second.htm

Bereavement Resources
Grief Recovery Institute: 8306 Wilshire Blvd., Los Angeles, CA 90211, Tel 213-650-1234, Hotline 800-445-4808 (hotline hours: 8:00 a.m.–5:00 p.m.) The National Grief Recovery Hotline seeks to ease the isolation of those suffering from a loss and assists them in coping with their grief.

Grief Recovery Online
Groww, Inc: 931 N. State Road 434, Ste. 1201-358, Altamonte Springs, FL 32714, Tel 407-865-9249. This is an independent haven for the bereaved developed by the bereaved–OUR PLACE. www.groww.com/

The Compassionate Friends Inc: P.O. Box 3696 Oak Brook, IL 60522-3696, Tel 630-990-0010. This is a national nonprofit, self-support organization which offers friendship and understanding to families who are grieving the death of a child of any age. www.compassionatefriends.org/

GriefNet, P.O. Box 3272, Ann Arbor, MI 48106-3272. This is a nonprofit corporation coming together and forming an Internet community consisting of more than 30 email support groups and two web sites. They provide support to people working through loss and grief issues of all kinds. www.griefnet.org/   E-mail Visibility@griefnet.org

California Consumer Health Care Council: This is an advocate for California health care consumers in all available forums. California Consumer Health Care Council, 200 Grand Avenue, #106, Oakland, CA 94610, Tel 510-419-0757, www.cchcc.org/

Health Administration Responsibility Project (HARP):
This site contains good information about health care policy and
HMOs as well as information about how to get legal help when
you've had a problem with your managed care plan. HARP, 552
12th St., Santa Monica, CA 90402-2908. www.harp.org/

Health on the Net: This is a vast, all-purpose medical reference
site. The medical community heavily uses it. C/O Medical
Informatics Division, University Hospital of Geneva, 1211 Geneva
14, Switzerland. www/hon/ch/ E-mail Info@hon.ch

Medicare HMOs: This site is exclusively dedicated to providing
extensive information about Medicare HMOs for anyone who is
considering joining one, or who is interested in getting additional information about them. www.medicarehmo.com
• ***Medicare Patients and Second Opinions Before Surgery***
   www.medicarenhic.com/bene/2ndopn.htm

Families' USA Foundation: Families USA is a national nonprofit, non-partisan organization dedicated to the achievement of
high-quality, affordable health and long-term care for all
Americans. Working at the national, state and community levels,
they have earned a national reputation as an effective voice for
health care consumers. 1334 G Street NW, Washington, D.C.
20005, Tel 202-628-3030. www.familiesusa.org/

Managed Care: This site includes information on how managed
care impacts children's health. 1935 Motor Street, Dallas, TX
75235, Tel 214-539-2576. www.childrens.com/mantop11.htm

Patient Advocacy Services: This site is to help consumers
reach a fair resolution of thjeir health insurance claim disputes or
denials. www.paidclaim.com/ E-mail info@paidclaim.com

The Center for Patient Advocacy: 1350 Bev erly Road, Suite
108, Mclean, VA 22101, Tel 703-748-0400 or 1-800-846-7444.
www.patientadvocacy.org/
• ***Checking Out Your Doctor:***
   www.patientadvocacy.org/main/checkout/

- *Medicare Issues:*
  www.patientadvocacy.org/main/medicare/agencies
- *The Patients' Bill of Rights Act:*
  www.patientadvocacy.org/main/managedcare/bora.htm
These sites represent the interest of patients nationwide.

***The National Coalition of Mental Health Professionals &
Consumers, Inc:*** This is a national organization of professional,
consumers, and consumer advocates. They are working to
address the negative impact of managed care on patients and
professionals in mental health care. The National Coalition, P.O.
Box 438, Commack, New York 11725, Tel 1-888-SAY-NO-MC
(1-888-729-6662) or 1-516-424-5232.
www.nomanagedcare.org/
- ***Rescue Health Care Day: April 1, 2000.*** All Americans
Concerned about Quality Health Care are invited to join in the
Nationwide Vote of "No Confidence" in Managed Care and the
National Dialogue on Alternatives to Managed Care. Why April
1st??? Because April 1st is April Fools Day and many Americans
feel they have been fooled by the promises of the managed care
industry. www.nomanagedcare.org/rhcd.htm
*Participate at any level in the Nationwide Day of Teach-Ins
Saturday, April 1, 2000*
Hour of Protest: 11:30 am–12:30 pm
Minute of Silence: 12:00 Noon
*For more information or to coordinate, contact the above
organization.*

***Members of The California State Medical Board–
1999/2000:*** Medical Board members are appointed by the
Governor (12 physicians and 5 public members), the Speaker of
the Assembly (1 public member), and the Senate Rules
Committee (1 public member). They serve a four-year term and
can be reappointed to a second term. Medical Board of
California, 1426 Howe Avenue, Suite 54, Sacramento, CA 95825-
3236, Tel 916-263-2389.
www.medbd.ca.gov/members.htm
- ***Other Health Professions:*** This is a list of people for consumers to contact when they have a problem with someone who

is not on the list of professionals the Board regulates.
www.medbd.ca.gov/otherprf.htm
- *Physician License Verification:*
  www.medbd.ca.gov/verifica.htm

American Board of Medical Specialties: This site will allow you to access their database to learn whether a physician is Board Certified in a specialty.
www.certifieddoctor.org

- *Diversion Program:* The Diversion program is administered by the Medical Board of California to monitor the recovery of physicians who have abused alcohol and/or drugs, or who have a mental or physical health problem which affects their ability to practice medicine safely.

ANYONE can urge a physician to contact the program, and can provide him or her the phone number. Tel 916-263-2600.
www.medbd.ca.gov/diverson.htm

Comments and Complaints: Consumers can contact the Board's Central Complaint Unit for assistance either through our tollfree line 1-800-633-2322 or by calling 916-263-2424.
www.medbd.ca.gov/complan1.htm

- *Important and Useful Phone Numbers:*
  www.medbd.ca.gov/phoenos.htm

NOTE: For all other States the resources are readily available. Your telephone directory will guide you to your local chapters and you will also find it on the Internet.

U.S. Government Advisory Panel: Janet Corrigan, Executive Director, Advisory Commission on Consumer Protecton and Quality in the Health Care Industry, 200 Independence Avenue, Hubert Humphrey Bldg., Room 118F, Washington, D.C. 20301. This panel is making rules about the HMO industry for the President and Congress to consider. These rules are supposed to protect you and your loved ones from unscrupulous HMO practices. Please make your views known by writing to the above address.

How to Contact Your State Senator: Office of Senator (name), United States Senate, Washington, D.C. 20510, Tel 202-224-3121. www.senate.gov/senators/index.cfm

How to Contact Your State Representative: United States House of Representatives, Washington, D.C. 20515, Tel 202-224-3121. www.house.gov/

The Ten Commandments for HMOs: If you're thinking of joining an HMO, or of changing from one HMO to another, send out the Ten Commandments for HMOs, plus the Questions to ask your HMO. Ask the HMO to respond with answers. If they don't answer, or if you don't like the answers, DON'T JOIN that HMO. Do the same with another HMO until you find one that answers your consumer concerns. When more people ask good questions and insist on answers, we'll have better consumer protection for everybody.

The Ten Commandments for HMOs

www.healthcare-disclose.com.

Prepared by Elizabeth Charlton Moore

lizmoore@healthcare-disclose.com

NOTE: Colorado is pioneer in requiring health insurance companies to provide extensive information to all potential policyholders. For more information write Colorado Division of Insurance, 1560 Broadway, Denver, CO 80202. Attention: Barbara Yondorf.

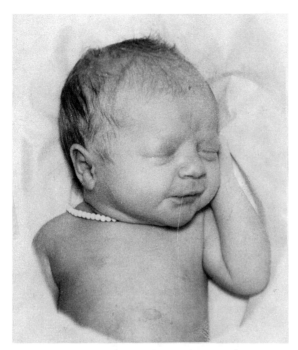

Jenny, 1 hour old, March 7, 1956

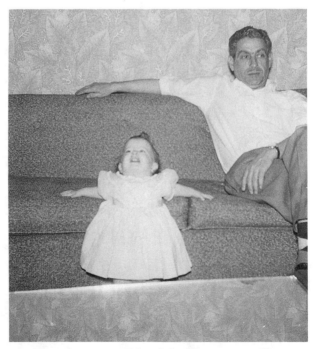

Jenny, age 1, and her father, Lucian Cancilla

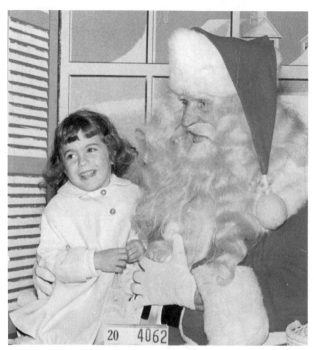

Jenny, age 3, with Santa, 1959

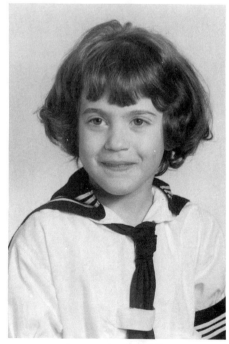

Jenny, age 6, 1961

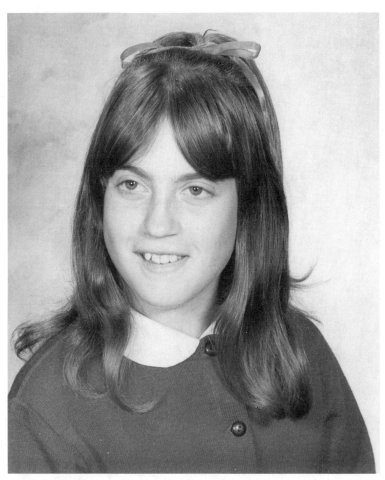

Jenny, 8 years old, 1963

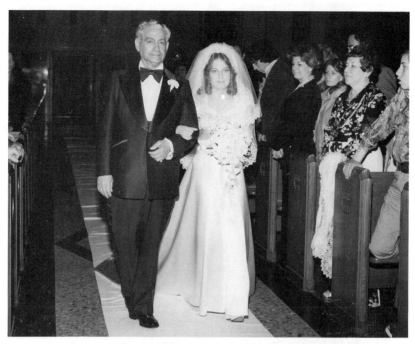

Jenny and her father, Wedding Day, March 19, 1977

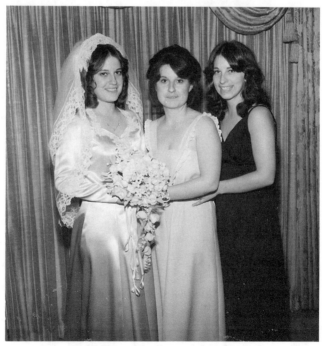

Jenny and her sisters, Rose and Cathy

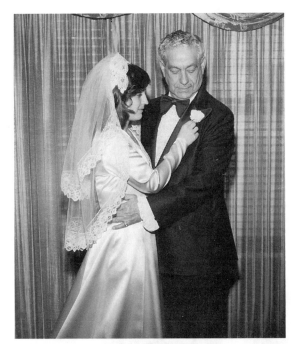

Jenny and her father

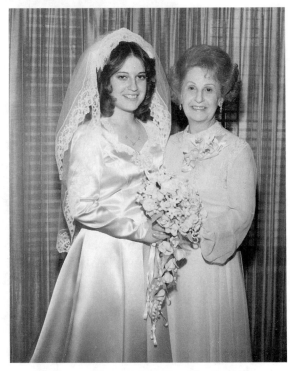

Jenny and her mother, Dorothy Cancilla

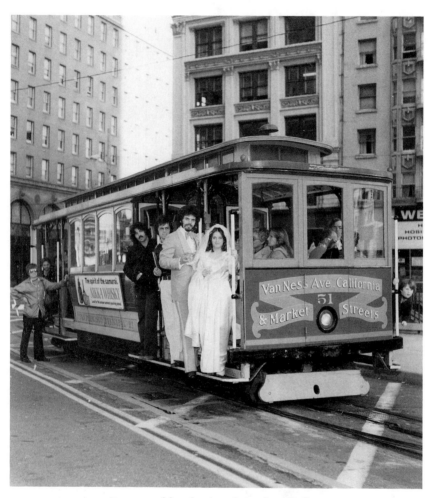

Jenny and her husband, Paul Gigliello,
in San Francisco on their Wedding Day, March 19, 1977

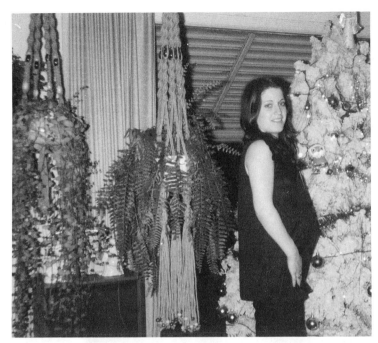

Jenny, 7 months pregnant, on Christmas Day, December, 1977

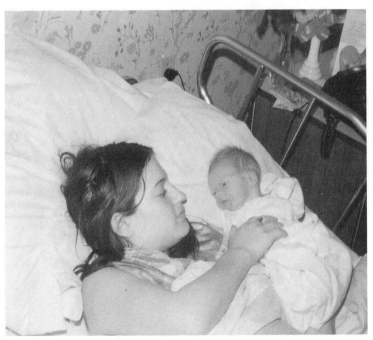

Jenny and her son, Paulie (Paul Jr.), 1 day old, March 11, 1978

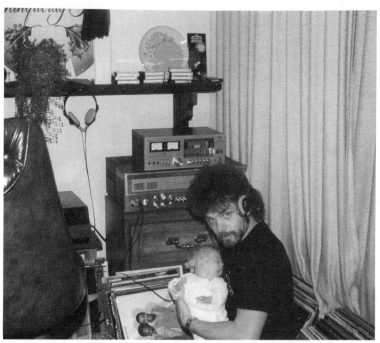

Paul Sr., with Paulie, at home, April, 1978

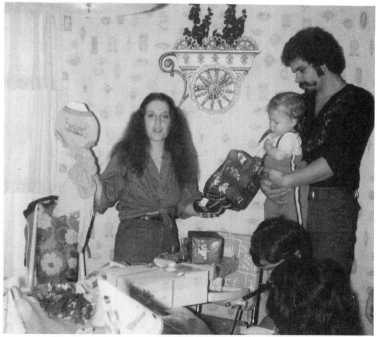

Jenny and Paul Sr., celebrating Paulie's 1st birthday

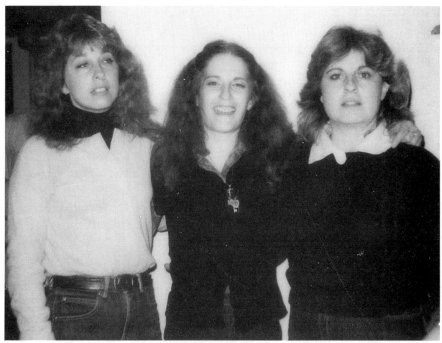

Jenny (middle) with her sisters Cathy (left) and Rose (right), while Jenny was being treated by Kaiser, 1985

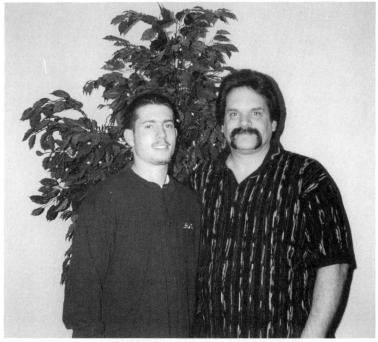

Paul Jr., with his father, Paul Sr., at home, April, 1999

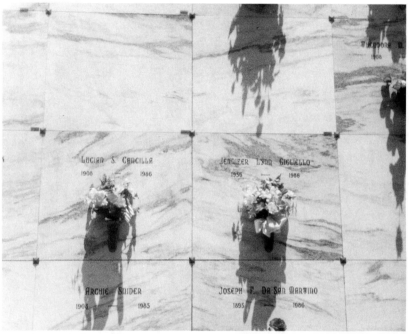

Jennifer Gigliello and her father, Lucian Cancilla, at their final resting place